THE
NIGHT
THE
LIGHTS
WENT
OUT

HARMONY BOOKS

NEW YORK

THE
NIGHT
THE
LIGHTS
WENT
OUT

DREW MAGARY

Copyright © 2021 by Drew Magary

All rights reserved.
Published in the United States by Harmony Books, an imprint of
Random House, a division of Penguin Random House LLC, New York.
harmonybooks.com

Harmony Books is a registered trademark, and the Circle colophon
is a trademark of Penguin Random House LLC.

Library of Congress Cataloging-in-Publication Data is available upon request.

ISBN 978-0-593-23271-2
Ebook ISBN 978-0-593-23272-9

Printed in the United States of America

Book design by Jen Valero
Jacket design by Pete Garceau
Jacket photograph: Elenathewise/iStock/Getty Images Plus

10 9 8 7 6 5 4 3 2 1

First Edition

For everyone you're about to meet within these pages

Some days
My brain
Blows up
In an elegant way

—BOB MOULD, 2019

CONTENTS

PART III

A NOTE FROM THE AUTHOR

Some names in this book have been changed. Many of the details are taken from medical records and interviews, but some are from my memory. Given that I am diagnosed amnesiac, you're gonna have to take your chances with me here.

Also, I've endeavored to make sure that everything I've written about my condition is as accurate as possible. If you have a problem with the medical details in this book, please call my office and schedule an appointment so I can have a look at it. I'll be sure to make you wait fifty minutes past that appointment time. Please note that I am an out-of-network author.

PROLOGUE

1984

This was gonna be a legit playdate. No bullshit. Mitch himself had invited me over personally. I was only in first grade, but that didn't stop me from being a social climber. Back in the eighties, you got tagged with that epithet at school if you were unrelentingly thirsty. But I wanted friends, and I wanted other kids to know that I had them. Was that so wrong?

In my mind, I was clearly different from the social climbers because I DESERVED more friends. All the other booger eaters deserved their place at the bottom of the grade-school clique system. Not me. This playdate with Mitch was gonna be my ticket to BMOC status. Kids were gonna consider themselves lucky to be *my* friend. They would beg me to come over to their place, and I would get to play with all of their toys, instead of playing with my own boring crap. I would be the king of Chicago.

So when Mitch asked me over, I pounced on his offer like it was a free Mrs. Fields cookie. We were gonna be Official Friends, which was a potential stepping-stone to acquiring more Official Friends. I needed those badly. I was *desperate* to be liked. This happens when you're a first grader, obviously. It also happens when you're an overweight loudmouth, which I also was at the time. I was picked last for games of dodgeball and for pretty much everything else as well. One time, at recess, Brian found a copy of *Playboy* sitting in a ditch. He let all the other boys have a look inside but didn't bother to offer me a turn. I guess he was doing me a favor, because whenever I saw bare boobs at age seven in a PG movie (just try watching an eighties PG movie with your kids now; the MPAA was a lot more forgiving back then), it freaked me out. That didn't stop dirty little Drew from wishing he had been worthy of a peek inside an honest-to-God porno mag, though. That desperation to be liked wouldn't subside for many, many years.

The day arrived. I went over to Mitch's apartment. I remember one thing that happened during the playdate and one thing only.

We were playing on the couch. If you know kids, you know that they don't treat furniture the way normal people treat furniture. You eat off a dining table; they carve pentagrams into it. You lovingly curate a collection of lamps and pretty pictures to adorn your side tables; they use those tables for storing Legos, Matchbox cars, Rubik's Cubes, and any other shit that they've gotten tired of playing with. You *sit* on a couch. No child has ever just sat on a couch. A whole new cycle of human evolution will have to pass before they do. To kids, a couch is a hiding spot, a chaise longue, a fort, a hurdle for show horses, a garbage can, a trampoline, and whatever the fuck else they feel like making it on a whim. If this were an ad, I would tell you that a couch is a fantastic blank canvas upon which a child can color in the farthest reaches of their imagination.

But this is not an ad. Mitch and I were not engaging in some spontaneous Montessori lesson. All we wanted to do was stand on top of the couch and wrestle. So we did.

As in any living room—all of which are uncomfortable and useless—there was a coffee table stationed in front of the couch, where grown-ups could rest their drinks and stack unread copies of *Time* magazine. I didn't notice this table, or its sharp corners, until it was too late. Mitch and I were standing on the couch and monkeying around when I lost my balance and fell backward. No way to break my fall. No way to turn around and brace myself. The back of my head smashed into one of the corners.

I'd had my share of boo-boos as a kid, but I had never required stitches for anything. I was gonna need stitches for this. Many of them. I felt something spongy and wet on the back of my head. *That's my brain,* I thought to myself. *My brain is coming out of me.* When I pulled my hand away, it was drenched in blood. I had no idea you could bleed that much and not die. A kid at school named Diego once bragged at lunchtime that he had tasted his own blood and that it tasted like grape juice. I now had what felt like a gallon of Welch's running down my wrist.

I screamed like a Mack truck drifting sideways down the highway. Mitch's face turned whiter than milk. His mom came running into the room. The playdate was over. I was going to the hospital.

My mom came and took me to the emergency room, where doctors laid me facedown on the bed and held me by my neck to keep me from moving. I was still screaming. I was not a kid who hid his emotions well. What you saw and heard from me was precisely what I was feeling. I made enough noise to let everyone in the OR, and probably greater Chicago, know that I was in shrieking pain. *I* could hear me. Primal screams flew out of my mouth, looped around my face, and flew back into my two pristine ears, scaring me shitless. The pain was the only thing I could hear. The metallic scent of my own coagulating blood was all I could smell.

The doctor begged me to calm down and told me that I would be all right. My brain was NOT coming out of my head, he assured me. I didn't believe him. As far as I was concerned, he had all the credibility of my mom in the driver's seat telling me that we were almost at the end of a long road trip. I knew this doctor was lying because he told me, "I'm going to stitch up your wound. It'll hurt"—say it with me—"*just a little bit.*"

"Are you gonna use a needle?" I asked him. I hated needles.

I'd had enough splinters before this injury to know that needles sucked.

"Yes, I'll use a needle."

"I DON'T WANNA SEE IT!"

"We're gonna numb up the area a little bit and you won't feel it much."

Again, lies. I felt the whole of the needle puncture my scalp again and again. Hurt just as much as if he hadn't used any anesthetic at all. The stitch job never ended. This was 1984, mind you. Today they could patch up a similar wound in half a second using Dermabond and surgical tape. But in 1984, I got the Civil War treatment. After an eternity of stabbing pain the doctor finished his gruesome handiwork and my mom took me home. At some point along the way, I transitioned from screaming to crying in staccato jags. My jacket became a bib for quick-spreading tears and snot.

Mitch never invited me over again.

After that, I took notice of tables anytime I encountered them. Mom did, too. We had a linoleum-covered table in the TV room with corners so sharp they could calve a fucking iceberg. If I ever got a little rambunctious within a mile of that table, Mom begged me to settle down. I don't know why she didn't just get rid of the thing. It's not like it was some priceless heirloom from czarist Russia. I think she got it at Caldor. Regardless, the table stayed, and I avoided it like it was a stranger with candy.

I never played on top of furniture ever again. Mom wouldn't let me and I didn't want to. I remained wary of sharp edges forever after that. When I eventually had kids of my own, my wife and I made sure all of our tables had rounded corners. Whenever our kids played at a house that hadn't been kid-proofed, I went full helicopter dad and monitored them if they were horsing around near glass furniture or other potential hazards. Then I'd complain about the setup on the ride home. *You see how sharp that table was? That table's a killer!*

Meanwhile, back in the eighties, I grew comfortable with my new battle wound. I liked to touch the scar. I liked telling other kids the story of how I got it, like I had gotten into a knife fight with a biker gang. It was just the right kind of scar. An ace up my sleeve. I could bust it out for special, buzz-cutty occasions, or I could easily keep it hidden. No one ever had to know it was there, or why.

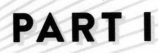

PART I

CHRISTMAS

2016

I needed a watch and a dog, in that order. It was Christmas and I was finally gonna get off my ass and buy a few Statement Gifts. Our three kids—Flora, Rudy, and Colin—had been bitching for a dog for two years. I stoically rebuffed them every time they made the request. I told them, "I'll think about it," which is boilerplate Dad-ese for NO. Interchangeable with "We'll see" as a cheap way to buy time while your kids walk away convinced that they've still got a chance at something. If I had said no outright to them, they would have dropped to the ground screaming and gone into exorcism convulsions, the way all kids do when they're denied something they want. Instead, I strung my kids along on the dog matter, like I was distracting them on a walk through the grocery store candy aisle.

I didn't want a dog. In my mind, I had graduated from caring for small things. Our three children were no longer babies. I was done with diapers. I was done with scrubbing Dr. Brown's formula bottles, breaking each one down into its thirty-seven constituent parts in the sink so I could pick out mildew from each part using a glorified pipe cleaner. Never again. I was free. I walked past newborn babies out in the wild and thought to myself, *Oh my God, that baby is so cute! Thank God we're never ever having one again!* In fact, I voluntarily paid a urologist to cut into my scrotum to ensure we wouldn't. After my vasectomy was over, the nurse discharging me told me, "Congratulations! Your family is complete!" Goddamn right it was, lady. We were finished. There would be five of us and no more.

That was where I stood. I was finished with small-mammal caregiving. Now these kids wanted us to adopt a fourth, very hairy baby that doesn't get any smarter and eats dried kangaroo pellets? Fuck no, man. That would cut into Daddy's beer time.

Of course, the story of any middle-aged dad is the story of a man vainly attempting to stand his ground while it shifts uncontrollably beneath him. The children persisted. They swore they'd take care of the dog. They'd feed it. They'd walk it, even in the rain. They'd housebreak it: a real leap of faith given how many years it took my wife, Sonia, and me to get those three kids to shit in a regulation toilet. I held firm. *No, no, no, no, we're good as is. If you guys need something that's yippy and shits a lot, Colin is right there.*

Alas, this was not solely my decision to make. Unlike me, Sonia grew up with a dog, and one day during the "Can we have a dog?" onslaught, she turned to me and was like, "You know, a dog could be really good for them."

That was it. Once the kids had Sonia in their pocket, it was all over.

My wife, as you will soon discover, possesses a tenacity that's far easier to submit to than to push back against. If she has an idea, she WILL see it through. If she asks me to do something and I take too long to get started on it for her liking, she bulls ahead and does it herself. The woman is a goddamn train. She and the kids worked me over as a team until Christmas crept over the horizon and I could see, with growing clarity, a vision of our kids bounding down the stairs Christmas morning and being greeted by a sprightly little doggy named Otis or Kirby or Biscuit or Cerberus wagging his tail and licking their faces.

I was in on the dog.

Timing-wise, a dog does not make an ideal Christmas-morning present, especially if you're intent on adopting one from a shelter and not from a breeder. You can't wrap it. You can't hide it in the basement for a month. If you bring a dog home late on Christmas Eve and stick it by the tree, it's not just gonna hang out there with a cup of hot cider and chill until the sun rises. Instead, this Christmas Eve, Santa wrote a letter to the kids consecrating the Future Acquisition of Dog. Sonia and I placed the letter on the living room coffee table—jumping near it not allowed—next to St. Nick's usual plate of unfinished, stale cookies. That was their statement present: Dad going from "I'll think about it" to "I have finally thought about it."

Meantime, I needed a watch. Sonia and I had been married for fourteen years and had settled into a place where we rarely, if ever, bothered to buy each other gifts for *any* occasion. Not for Christmas. Not for birthdays. Definitely not for Valentine's Day. There were a lot of reasons for this, chief among them the fact that we were cheap and lazy. We knew that we had to save every dollar we earned during the kids' upbringing so that, once they turned college age, the nefarious debt lords at BIG UNIVERSITY could extinguish our life savings in half a second. I worked as a sports blogger for Deadspin at the time: a dream job in many ways, but not necessarily in salary. I made good money, but not tens of millions of dollars. So there was no dough available to fritter away on a countertop bread maker or some other perfunctory Christmas gift that adults get tired of more quickly than children do of their gifts.

Besides, we both preferred homemade gifts from the kids: handprints, notes, pictures of Transformers that Colin made me print out so he could color them in, sloppy collages, etc. Gifts like these are living artifacts of your kid's personality, and of that exact moment in their life, in a way that nothing from a store can be. I would not be able to remember what Flora was like at age five without her works from that era. I papered the walls of my home office with all of these gifts, to remind myself who I really worked for. Years later, I would remove that artwork and replace it with a single framed, collective art project of theirs that means more to me than anything else I own.

The downside of all that syrupy perspective was that it rendered both Sonia and me stereotypical "Oh, I don't need anything" parents who are annoyingly difficult to shop for. For her part, Sonia enjoyed returning things much more than she enjoyed buying them. So it felt wasteful to buy each other gifts that would prove either useless or burdensome. Instead, we just bought shit for ourselves as needed. One time I bought myself a smoker that retroactively became my Father's Day gift two months later. I smoked enough ribs to make your heart choke.

You can call this a rut, but it was an awfully comfortable one. Sonia and I were confident in our routine. We knew each other well enough to know what we needed and when we needed it. There was no need (or cash) for me to go all out and show up with a fucking Lexus in the driveway on Christmas morning, a haughty yuppie bow glued to the top of it. I only needed to get Sonia a big Christmas present if the stars aligned and there was something cool she needed right when the holidays came around.

Luckily for me, her watch had become a piece of shit.

Through the early years of our marriage, Sonia relied on a Swiss Army watch her parents had given her for her high school graduation. This watch sucked its battery dry with gluttonous efficiency. She got the battery swapped out every four months, trudging down to a local watch repair shop that fulfilled every idea you have in your mind about what a local watch repair shop looks like. You walk in the door and you're greeted by the sight of a thousand old clocks and other assorted curios, all gathering dust. The proprietor, a very nice man, owns a parrot that hangs out on the counter, its talons long enough to dig a trench across your brain. This is the kind of shop that may or may not have a portal to a witch's cottage in the back. An old lady is always waiting in front of you in line, and she's never there for a routine watch job. No, no, she came because she needs the pallet bridge inside an antique pocket watch removed, soaked in gold leaf, buffed to a high gloss, lacquered in TruCoat, and then reinstalled inside a *different* watch she got for eight bucks at the estate sale of a dead neighbor.

Sonia would get her battery replaced, wear it home, pray it stayed alive, and then cry out, "IT'S BROKEN AGAIN!" months later. But she loved the watch, so much so that she bought me my own Swiss Army watch back in 2000. It was a splurge for her, given what we were making at the time. She told me after the fact, "I bought that watch because I was like, *This guy is the one. At least, he better be.*"

I was. We got married in 2002, with matching watches to boot. When you're married, you gotta be real careful about matching. If you dress exactly the same, you look like the stars of a fucking nursery rhyme. Matching watches were a touch more discreet. People might notice we were wearing the same watch, but we weren't clad in identical gingham bonnets or anything. We were a tastefully, harmoniously accessorized couple.

Sadly, I wasn't long for my watch. I had a terrible habit of losing watches and sunglasses, so I never bought expensive ones. When I was a kid, my folks got me an Ironman watch, making me a certified triathlete. I lost it while swimming in the Atlantic. Years after that, they bought me a nicer watch. A legit watch. That one lasted a few weeks before I bumped against a support beam in Grand Central station and never saw it again. My mom demanded I go to the Grand Central lost and found to recover it. Did you know that Grand Central has a lost and found? It's like going to a car impound.

Now I had a watch that was not only pricey but also a token of Sonia's love for me. Her faith in me. I was terrified of losing it. One time its crown came spinning off and I nearly had a breakdown. Also, I had an iPhone, which made wearing watches redundant.

So one night I left the watch in a drawer in my nightstand and left it there for years, next to a couple of stray books. The battery inside that watch of mine died. I rarely, if ever, wore it after that. But at least I knew where it was. It was safe in my drawer. Protected.

Now Sonia's own watch was failing her. I made a plan. I took Flora aside.

"I wanna get Mom a watch for Christmas. Can you help me?"

"Do we need to go to the mall to find it?" Flora loved the mall.

"Yeah."

"YES!"

Off we went. She was only ten at the time, but Flora had already become a discerning shopper. When kids are younger than that, they want you to buy them shit just so that they can have it. But Flora was well past that stage. She had a few twenties in her wallet but wouldn't spend her loot on just anything. Whatever she bought had to fit into her now-established style, which usually involved a hoodie of some sort. This was the kind of shrewd retail mind I required. My goal was to buy my wife something that she wouldn't return, or would return only with pained reluctance.

The plan was to stick exclusively to solar-powered watches. No battery. No trips to the watch store to get one replaced. No parrot asking for a cracker before it squawks, "YOU'RE FAT!" at you.

Flora and I walked into Macy's at the local mall and browsed the counter. Do you know how strange it is to ogle a department store jewelry counter with the actual INTENT to buy something? I felt like a billionaire. When the woman behind the counter asked me if I needed assistance, I actually said yes. I never say yes to these people. I normally run away from them screaming, like they're a window salesman trying to hand me a flyer.

Flora and I found a watch. Tasteful. Elegant. Not terribly expensive (phew!), and powered by the mighty sun. We took it home and I wrapped it. I am never in charge of Christmas wrapping in the Magary household. This is less because of my dadly sloth, though that almost certainly factors in, and more because I am ill-equipped for the task. There were certain chores that Sonia had banned me from doing because I sucked so deeply at them. Folding laundry was one. Decorating was another. Wrapping presents was perhaps my greatest Achilles' heel. It looks like I did it with my teeth.

This time, I cut the paper cleanly, made atomically precise creases, and taped it together with all the effort and care that Sonia deserved. Maybe she'd hate the watch, but by God she'd RESPECT the way it had been lovingly enveloped in a swatch of Target-brand snowman paper.

And she did respect it. She still returned it, of course, but she found another solar-powered beauty at the same Macy's counter and in the same price range. I had not gotten her the correct gift, but I had gotten the correct parameters for a gift. Close enough! Everyone won. I could hear the appreciation in Sonia's voice when she opened it that Christmas morning. It was legit. In return, she got me booze. The perfect default gift. I loved booze and wasn't fussy about it. No need to ever return any. I think I got new grill tongs, too. Useful for the Father's Day smoker.

This decidedly romantic gift exchange between Sonia and me

happened well after the kids had rushed downstairs and read the Dog Letter out loud to one another to confirm what it entailed. Santa also got them some doggy toys in advance. That way they knew it wasn't just horseshit.

"We're really getting a dog?" Rudy asked.

"Yeah!" I said.

"Can we go get one now?" Flora asked.

"Well, nowhere is open right now. You will have to wait a bit."

That answer was too close to a "We'll see" for Flora's taste. She was not interested in waiting a bit. No more stalling. In an instant, she was on PetConnect searching for shelter dogs nearby and falling in love with every thumbnail. Within two days, she had found a couple of adoption candidates that fit all of our criteria. They were small. They were cute. They had no criminal record. They were relatively close by. So, on New Year's Eve morning, we hopped into our white minivan, featuring an exterior made of Tupperware, and drove across the Potomac to a no-kill shelter in Virginia. I reminded the kids that this was a process. We were probably gonna have to visit *many* shelters to find the exact dog we wanted. Another standard parent move: the pre-letdown. They had no interest in tempering their expectations. They wanted the new dog that Santa had promised them. Right now.

Once inside the shelter, we were greeted by a squall of locked-up dogs barking with maximum friskiness. They were scared. They were irritable. They were excited. They were hungry. The place smelled like an armpit factory. We met a dog on Flora's list named Cookie. A brown dog. Cookie was kind of a dick. We were disappointed. Looking for a new dog is like shopping for a car. You hope that the one you had your eye on turns out to be the one. Cookie was not the one.

But Cookie wasn't the *only* dog at the shelter. There were more dogs out in an adjacent play yard, including Carter, whose thumbnail Flora had also bookmarked. Carter's profile stated that he was three years old and potentially a mix of Shih Tzu, Maltese, and poodle. A shitpoo. The copy read: "Carter loves toys. Did we mention that Carter loves toys? Carter LOVES toys." Sounded like he'd fit right in with this lot.

More prospective dog owners packed into the shelter to snoop around. We had competition. One of the workers took us into the yard and there, on the opposite side of a chain-link fence, was Carter. The worker grabbed him and brought him over to the kids. He sniffed their faces. They giggled. He licked Colin's eyelid.

"Carter, you're crazy!"

That was it. The kids were playing with Carter like they had always owned him. We were walking to the office to sign his adoption papers before I could even process that this was going down.

"So I guess we're getting this dog?" I asked Sonia.

"We're getting a dog!"

"Holy shit."

We paid the adoption fee and bought a care package for Carter that included a crate, a leash, a harness, and a nine-hundred-pound bag of dry food that he ended up hating. An old lady walked past the cashier's desk and asked to see Carter, but we had already staked our claim to him. I felt awful we beat her, though not awful enough to give him up.

We loaded Carter into our marshmallow van for the half-hour drive back home. I was worried he'd piss all over the car, but Carter was too freaked out about being driven to Maryland by a bunch of strange white people to rip out a stream. The doggy adrenaline kept his walnut bladder in check. The kids voted to keep his shelter name (the shelter rep said he'd answer to any new name, provided you had a treat in your hand when uttering it). Sonia and I agreed. Otherwise, the kids would have just fought for a month over what to name him and landed on something worse, like Huckleturd or something.

We got home. Carter bounded into the house, rocketing toward every toy the kids sent him to fetch. The PetConnect page wasn't lying. My man really did love toys. This playdate was going marvelously. We brought Carter upstairs for his first bath, keeping the water shallow, just like when you wash a newborn. Sonia used the detachable showerhead to rinse months of captivity off of him. With wet fur, he looked half his weight. The kids toweled Carter off, stealing a moment to nuzzle against him on every pass. An hour later, he was presentably fluffy. He smelled fresh, too. He still smelled like a dog, but that was okay. I liked smelling dogs. Smelling is investigating. Dogs know this innately. Humans tend to forget the sense's established purpose.

Carter had huge eyes. You couldn't lie to those eyes. When he looked at us, it was like he was saying, *Hey, the fuck is going on here?* We had all the time in the world to explain it to him. He was one of us. *Now* our family was complete. As with having children, the moment you get a dog it seems unfathomable that you ever lived your life without one.

"This truly was the best Christmas ever," I told the kids. Another standard dad maneuver. Every Christmas is the best Christmas ever. But this time, I meant it. I had the dog and the gift receipt for a midrange watch to prove it. The kids nodded in vigorous assent. And things were only going to get better from here. My luck—*our* luck, really—promised only more adventures, more stability, and more rowdy love between the six of us.

Two years later, the solar battery in Sonia's new watch died. And so did I.

COLLAPSE

DECEMBER 2018

'll start with what I remember. I was in New York the night of December 5. I was there with all of my Deadspin co-workers for the Deadspin Awards at Irving Plaza. These were gag awards we handed out in prestigious categories such as Ass Team of the Year, and I was the host. Nominees were invited but never attended, which was how we preferred it. Really, this was a party. I had spent my early career working as an advertising copywriter, then switched over to *writing* writing as a full-time job in 2012, when Deadspin formally added me to its masthead. It was my favorite website in the world, and the people working there were my favorite people in the world. They were my best friends. I didn't wanna live without them.

Of course, the majority of them lived in New York, whereas I was now a family man bunkered down in suburban Maryland with Sonia, the kids, and Carter. My comfortable rut. Over the course of the decade, Deadspin grew more popular, eventually averaging tens of millions of unique visitors a month. But all of that success was online. I never got to see our burgeoning readership, nor many of the colleagues I spent every day with, in person. So this night wasn't just some rote off-site meeting. It was a rare moment to see, hear, feel, and even smell the fruits of my labor: readers packing the hall to see us in person, me standing up on a stage delivering one-liners à la Stephen Colbert, and me and my colleagues celebrating in person instead of inside a chat room. It was gonna be a fucking RAGER, man. Now in my forties, I had to portion out my late nights like they were army rations. This night, I would get to feast.

I was wearing a rented tux but not my watch. Before the show, I FaceTimed with Sonia to say good night to her and the kids, treating them to a glorious panorama of an at-the-moment empty ballroom. I don't remember anything I said to her, and neither does she. All I remember is that it was a routine check-in. *Hey! How are you? Did you guys have a good day at school? Oh, everything here is great! It's gonna be a blast. I probably won't be able to call you later because this place'll be too noisy. Love you!* I know we exchanged "I love yous" because that was how we ended every call. This wasn't a practice I grew up with. But when I was in college, I noticed that my best friend Howard's family always said it to each other while goodbye-ing, because it's a nice thing to hear from your family, no matter when or if you hear from them again.

So I stole it.

The doors to Irving Plaza opened and ticketholders flooded in to see me, the rest of the Deadspin staff, and a mascot named Shitty pretend to flush awards down a demo toilet. The crowd quickly cashed in their drink tickets and got loaded. Their collective excitement crept into the dressing room, growing stronger as showtime grew closer. I was lying down on the couch, to preserve my energy and rest my back. I tried to sneak in a nap but the excitement from outside was too contagious for me to pull one off. I liked it loud. I liked being in the middle of a bigass commotion, and often being the source of that commotion. I worked every day from home, where it got noisy only when Rudy and Colin got into a slapping war. I didn't normally get to hold court over a room of boisterous adults. So I cherished, with great zeal, the few occasions I got the opportunity.

Other Deadspin staffers went to grab drinks from the bar, but I abstained. This was rare for me. When I hosted this show in previous years, I always helped myself to a cocktail or three beforehand. My reasoning was that the booze would loosen me up and help shake off the nerves. The reality was that I just wanted to drink. Drinking was my preferred hobby. But I knew I'd be a better host this time around if I wasn't drinking on the job. Also, I was still getting over a nasty cold. The only thing I was high on during my monologue was a Z-Pak.

The show went off seamlessly. I made a glorious ass of myself onstage, all in accordance with the script. The crowd headed for the exits as our time as kings and queens of Irving Plaza came to an end. I slipped out the back door with my colleague Lauren Theisen and a friend of hers. From the club, the three of us walked four and a half blocks to a karaoke bar. That's a short distance as New York City walks go, except when it's cold as shit outside and you think the bar is closer than it actually is. I was looking forward to this after-party, probably more than the original awards show. I loved singing while getting hammered. I had a whole repertoire of songs in my head that I was gonna tear through. Would any of my friends enjoy hearing my drunken rendition of "Song 2" by Blur? No. But that didn't stop me from thinking they would. I quickened my step.

We got to the bar, where my boss, Megan Greenwell, had rented out a room downstairs. Her husband, Dr. David Heller, was already belting out "Reptilia" on the karaoke machine when we walked in. A bucket of beers arrived in our wake, along with the rest of our friends and colleagues. Victor Jeffreys, who essentially produced the entire awards show, arrived carrying a big stack of pizza boxes. The person who brings the pizza to the party is always the hero. I warmed up my pipes with "You Got Lucky," by Tom Petty, which soon would prove either fitting or ironic, depending upon your perspective. I have no idea why I picked this song. I had never sung it at a karaoke bar before. It was just floating through my mind and I grabbed it.

There weren't enough people in the room yet for me to bring the house down with classic dad rock, but I enjoyed my first turn at the mic. It was a proper warm-up. I crammed down a slice of pizza for energy, grabbed a well-deserved Miller Lite, and then walked out of the room into the hallway—a very dark hallway lined with bare concrete—to take a piss.

That's when I collapsed.

THE WITNESSES

THE NIGHT OF DECEMBER 5

The next thing I remember is waking up in a hospital bed, groggily watching doctors, nurses, and my family as they passed through my line of vision, seemingly at random. I was in an ICU. No more tux. There were tubes running out of every part of me, an IV jammed into my wrist, and a CPAP stuffed up my nostrils. I felt around my head and, yep, there were tubes coming out of there as well. There was also a catheter inside my penis.

I had no idea what was wrong with me. There was no pain emanating from any specific part of my body. I remembered I was at the karaoke bar and singing my little song. After that came a great void. The good news was that I knew I was me. I was Drew Magary. I was married to Sonia. My kids were Flora, Rudy, and Colin. We lived in Maryland. I wrote for a living. I loved banana pudding. All of that was still there. Check, check, check.

I figured that it was the following day, December 6. My brother Alex's birthday. I also figured that I had gotten into a fistfight with someone and lost. I had a train home to catch that morning. Now I'd missed it. *Fuck*. And the party! I'd missed the whole goddamn after-party, too. That was even more annoying. I never got to sing the Blur song! Everyone would have gone WILD for it.

A kind nurse clarified the situation for me. I had not gotten into a fistfight. I had inexplicably fainted in that lounge hallway. On my way to the ground, I fractured the temporal bone in my skull because, once again, I had no way to brace myself for the impact. This was the first bone I'd ever broken in my life, and I picked a fucking doozy. The temporal bone is the hardest bone in the human body. To fracture it, you usually have to be assaulted, crash your car, or get shot. Or you could fall down and smash your head against a concrete floor. That might do the trick.

Also, the nurse told me, it was not December 6. It was December 19. I had been in a medically induced coma for two weeks. The world had gone missing to me, and I to it. I was not here. But everyone I cared about was.

So, for this part of the story, let me put you in their hands. This is eyewitness testimony from my friends, my family, my surgeon, and the Deadspinners who rushed to save my life that night. These are their words, as told to me for this book. Because this is their story as much as it is my own. I had the luxury to sleep through all of this. They did not.

MEGAN GREENWELL (editor in chief, Deadspin): Before the Deadspin Awards show, you asked for Advil. Either your head or your back was hurting you.

VICTOR JEFFREYS (colleague): You were in your tuxedo before the show, lying down on the couch. You were definitely quiet. More quiet than usual, maybe.

BARRY PETCHESKY (deputy editor, Deadspin): You were absolutely yourself that night. The pink of health.

HOWARD (my best friend): You were definitely in host mode at the show. You had a few drinks after, but as someone who's known you for the better part of twenty-five years, it was definitely not on the upper end of a big night out for Drew, at least up until that point. You were high energy, but you weren't strange at all. You were telling me you were amped up.

JESSE (also my best friend): I had been to a bunch of these Deadspin Awards in the past in shittier locations, but this was by far the most polished. You were in your tux, laughing it up, basking in the adulation of the Deadspin crew, lead singer of the rock band, and truly at the height of your powers.

And Howard says to me at one point, "Look at him up there. Aren't you so proud of him?"

MATT UFFORD (friend, former colleague): I was sad to miss the show because it was always a pretty good time and a chance to see you in your tuxedo and being the only person taking the dress code seriously.

JESSE: This one guy, long hair with a beard, I think, did give you a bag of weed candy that his girlfriend made for you. And you were like, "Thanks, man."

Howard and I look at you, flabbergasted. Howard's like, "You going to eat those?" And you're like, "Probably." And we're like, "All right, good luck, man." You put it in your pocket. You were saving it for later.

I never ended up consuming that weed candy, although I would have eaten it if I'd had the chance. It was almost certainly still inside the breast pocket of my rental tux when Victor Jeffreys returned it on my behalf after the accident.

CHRIS THOMPSON (writer, Deadspin): Maybe fifteen minutes after we arrived at the karaoke place, my wife, my sister, and I had a short interaction with you. You could not string together a sentence. You chugged most of a full beer and then wandered off. You seemed to go from happy drunk to disconcertingly hammered in a short period of time, so it seems likely it wasn't just the alcohol.

You and my wife had a brief exchange where you joked that she'd jumped in front of you in the karaoke order. It was during this song—maybe two minutes after that exchange, and maybe seven minutes after you'd chugged the beer—that you collapsed in the hallway.

BOBBY SILVERMAN (writer, Daily Beast): I realized I was down to my last cigarette. So I leave and there was a corridor that separated the main bar from the karaoke room. I could see a silhouetted figure on the right, standing but using the wall to stay upright. I walk over, I see you wearing the tuxedo. It was like you were falling asleep or really tired or inebriated, but I didn't know. I said something like *Hey, Drew, are you okay?* And you said, *Yeah, yeah, yeah, I'm fine.* Your face was pale. You were very sweaty. I certainly didn't see a head injury, but your head was pressed against the back wall. I wouldn't have been able to see it.

Your eyes were sort of closed. I said to you, *I can call a cab.* And you said, *No, no, no, no, I'm fine.* You also joked about "not being a kid anymore." And I said, *Okay, man, listen, just take care of yourself.*

JORGE CORONA (creative producer, Deadspin): From the corner of my eye, I see you in the hallway and I acknowledged subconsciously, *Oh, that's Drew.* And then I remember turning away. Maybe I took a bite of pizza or something. Way less than a minute. Ten seconds, I think. And then all of a sudden I felt a thud. Sometimes you *feel* through the noise.

I look over and you were on the ground. I noticed it more than anybody else around me would have. I was in the right spot, and the right sequence of events happened for me to have seen that right away.

KIRAN CHITANVIS (video director, Deadspin): I was just inside of the door when you collapsed. Jorge was next to me. He pulled open the door to see you on the floor, then immediately grabbed me and dragged me into the hallway.

JORGE CORONA: I was like, *We need to call an ambulance.*

KIRAN CHITANVIS: I saw you, then I came back inside the room to get my phone and immediately called 9-1-1. This is the first time I'd ever called 9-1-1.

MEGAN GREENWELL: Kiran came back in and it was very loud because people were singing karaoke. I didn't know exactly what she was communicating, but she clearly looked freaked out. Stricken.

SAMER KALAF (news editor, Deadspin): It was a bizarre situation because there was this very serious thing going on, and the people singing obviously had no idea what had happened.

KIRAN CHITANVIS: Victor had gone to get *more* pizzas for everybody. So he had just walked in, in the middle of all of this with, like, ten pizzas.

VICTOR JEFFREYS: When I came back with the pizza in hand, I turned the corner and Kiran looked at me. She goes, *There's been an accident.* I put the pizza down, walked another five feet, and you were right there. In that little hall.

JORGE CORONA: I went over to you. You had fallen onto your back, which was strange. Your hands came up to your chest. They curled up so that your wrists were almost touching your shoulders. That's when I was like, *Something is wrong.* That was the moment where I saw blood behind your head. It was thick. Slick, deep blood.

BARRY PETCHESKY: There was a big patch of blood. Maybe as wide as a dollar bill. It was *thick.* Not just, like, a light smear. I asked Jorge stupidly, *Is that blood?*

KIRAN CHITANVIS: Your eyes were open and your hands were tucked in a stressor position. Imagine if someone is paralyzed and they can't use their arms, but their fists are clenched.

BARRY PETCHESKY: Megan and I were worried, but we didn't realize how bad it was. We thought you had slipped and hit your head. We thought you had a concussion, which sucks. But like, it's a concussion. It was, *Oh shit, we can't just have a normal night out without one thing going to hell.*

KIRAN CHITANVIS: Your eyes were open and twitchy. You were not cognitive. You were not present. I know enough about minor injuries from having played sports over the years, and I've had enough concussions to know this was way worse.

SAMER KALAF: I was inside the karaoke room and (Deadspin writer) Laura Wagner was near the door, looking out the window. Her face was very severe. Pale. I saw for myself that you were in severe distress and then I was like, *I don't know what to do now. I don't want to be at karaoke and I don't want to eat pizza and I don't really want to talk to anybody.*

KIRAN CHITANVIS: Somewhere around that time you were sitting up and singing along to the song that was playing in the background, but the words were extremely slurred. I don't remember which song.

SAMER KALAF: At the time, Gabe and somebody else were performing the Afroman song ["Because I Got High"]?

LAUREN THEISEN: Oh, that was Gabe and Patty [Deadspin writer Patrick Redford]. For some reason I remember that clearly.

GABE FERNANDEZ (writer, Deadspin): I was singing along in a group. I had no clue you collapsed until the absolute end of the night. You mentioned you queued up "The Gambler" at one point. I remember singing that song in your place because you weren't in the room. I grabbed the mic because I knew the song and no one claimed it at the time.

KIRAN CHITANVIS: And then there was, like, *profuse* vomiting.

ALBERT BURNEKO (writer, Deadspin): I missed the fall itself, which is agonizing to think about because I couldn't have been more than maybe ten feet from where it happened. I heard groaning, and it took me a minute to separate it from all the other voices and sounds. Then I was like, "Oh shit, maybe somebody is having a hard time in this hallway," and I got up to check.

You were on the ground. I saw the blood and I saw vomit. A thing that never occurred to me before just now is that . . . maybe not all the vomit was yours? Maybe you could have slipped on somebody else's vomit and hit your head on the way down?

SAMER KALAF: You started throwing up a lot of blood. I guess I'm not positive if it was blood or not, but it definitely was not vomit. Either a dark red or a black.

MEGAN GREENWELL: As far as I know, you never vomited anything besides food and bile. Never saw any blood.

BARRY PETCHESKY: It was very thick throw-up, definitely like you had had food recently.

MEGAN GREENWELL: We were afraid you were going to choke on vomit. We were trying to turn your head to the side so that you didn't choke. There was vomit all over your tux and you said, *Oh fuck, this is a rental tux.*

BARRY PETCHESKY: I was kneeling oblique to you: one hand supporting your back, the other one in front of you. You splashed vomit everywhere. Up to midcalf on my leg.

ALBERT BURNEKO: You were conscious but you were also *gone,* you know what I mean?

BARRY PETCHESKY: You were nonsensical. You were trying to make words, but they were not intelligible.

JORGE CORONA: I was kneeling by your head. I pressed a towel behind your head, because I kept seeing blood coming out from in between your follicles. It just kept coming. I was trying to give you words of reassurance, which must have been really funny because nothing was okay about this.

BARRY PETCHESKY: At some point a bartender there got involved and she was EMS certified. She seemed very confident and in control. Very old business. *Keep him awake and talking.* She got you into the main entrance area. We all thought it was important to get you sitting up. So it was a multiperson operation to get you onto a couch.

MEGAN GREENWELL: I was saying to [my husband], even before the paramedics got there, *I don't think he's drunk.* You had one beer at Irving Plaza. And then you had one beer at the karaoke bar. The beers were in these buckets, and they were coming out so slowly that most people hadn't even gotten their hands on it.

DR. DAVID HELLER (internist, Mount Sinai Hospital, husband of Megan): I definitely noticed the blood. Whenever somebody has a nasty blow to the head that involves bleeding, it is rule number one of medicine that you always get a CT scan of their head as soon as possible, because there is a remote chance that they have a serious head bleed.

BARRY PETCHESKY: It took paramedics something like fifteen minutes to get there, which felt like an eternity at the time.

KIRAN CHITANVIS: The EMTs seemed convinced, regardless of the blood and everything like that, that you were just very drunk. They tried to stand you up and make you walk out. They got you three steps out of the hallway and into that main room. You keeled over sideways onto a banquette, slurring your words and not cognizant. Megan threw a fit to get them to strap you onto a gurney.

MEGAN GREENWELL: I'm like, *Dude, you can't make him walk.* David was trying to, like, doctor-reason with them, but I was just yelling.

DR. DAVID HELLER: I think I agreed with them that you were drunk, which proved incorrect, but I disagreed with how they were manhandling you. They were intending to take you to the hospital, but they were not under the impression that you were in need of it.

SITTING IN DREAD

SHORTLY AFTER MIDNIGHT, DECEMBER 6

Victor accompanied me in the back of the ambulance to Beth Israel Hospital downtown. Megan Greenwell and Dr. David Heller followed behind in a cab.

VICTOR JEFFREYS: I remember a lackadaisical attitude around the paramedics. *Oh, we see this a thousand times.* They hadn't even moved the fucking ambulance. I'm like, *Drive the goddamn thing! Don't you see something is wrong?*

I kept begging you for your fucking phone passcode. You would give me numbers. I tried every fucking combination of the thing. Nothing.

MEGAN GREENWELL: You thought you were being the class clown.

VICTOR JEFFREYS: You were saying things like *It hurts*, but yelling them. Then you would mumble. And you were throwing up. One time there was black stuff and another time it was, like, green.

JORGE CORONA: We were standing on the street outside the lounge, shocked, as a group.

KIRAN CHITANVIS: I remember someone handing me a whole pizza and being like, *Just take it home.* So I'm standing on a street corner in a gown, holding a pizza box. I get home and I realize that my shoes are caked in blood.

JORGE CORONA: I headed home with this weird sense of *What just happened? What can I do? What* did *I do just now?* I got home at like 2:00 A.M. and scrolled through Instagram. For a good hour. I was trying to distract myself without knowing that that's what I was doing.

BARRY PETCHESKY: I took a cab home and I went to sleep. I thought it was still going to be a concussion. I was going to wake up in the morning, you were going to be fine, and we were going to laugh about it.

When I woke up, I had a ton of missed calls and texts from Megan on my phone. Seeing the texts, I felt extremely guilty that I had not woken up.

MEGAN GREENWELL: Samer texted me to ask if we needed anything. I said no, but he showed up anyway with snacks.

SAMER KALAF: I went to Walgreens in Union Square and I got some Gatorade and candy. Megan and Victor were at the hospital with you. I knew if I went home, I would be sitting in that dread. And I was like, *It'll be like a nice thing to cheer him up when he wakes up, getting him some snacks.*

MEGAN GREENWELL: You saw us eating some candy and were mad you couldn't have some, which was fair.

VICTOR JEFFREYS: Megan and her husband got to the hospital *faster* than the ambulance. They got there way before we did. They probably got there before the ambulance left the fucking bar.

MEGAN GREENWELL: I pulled up LexisNexis on my phone to try to find your home number, but you fuckers don't have a landline. The quest for your phone passcode and/or Sonia's number went on for HOURS. We were trying some wild things. We called Gizmodo Media Group HR in the middle of the night. We scoured Facebook. We looked for Montgomery County PTA lists. And we argued with you for SO LONG about what your code was.

DR. DAVID HELLER: I was like, *All we have to do is get a CT scan. As long as there's no brain bleed, whatever this is, it should be fine.*

SAMER KALAF: You were talking in slow motion at some points. You were whimpering in a way that I had never heard from you before, pleading with nurses to be careful. Not in a way where you were telling the hospital staff what to do, but in a way where you were very vulnerable. You were whimpering and talking about how everything hurt.

It was one of the worst moments of my life. I feel, like, grateful to have had a life where I haven't had many terrible moments. This was definitely one of them: seeing somebody in severe distress and not being able to do anything about it.

> *Meanwhile, while all of this was happening, Sonia and the children were still all sound asleep back at our house in Maryland.*

SONIA (my wife): You went for a CT scan because Megan pushed for it. You know, they tried to turn you away and send you home. Megan's insistence that they examine you closer is what kept you alive.

SAMER KALAF: Megan and Victor were devastated, but they were definitely alert and agitating for more attention to you. I might've tried to say a few words to you, but I was mostly silent because I was just speechless.

MEGAN GREENWELL: The doctors and nurses were being so blasé about it, I started to doubt myself and I was like, *Okay, maybe he is drunk.*

You were trying to stand up and jump off of this hospital bed. I was trying to *stop* you from doing that. I was saying, *It's fine. We're just going to lie here for a few minutes. We're going to get to go home pretty soon.* You started getting agitated out of nowhere and fighting me. You were going downhill fast, thrashing up against me. I was using all of my body weight to try to hold you down, and it wasn't going well.

Right in that moment they got the CT scan results and everything went to a hundred. They were like, *He needs to be in the ICU right away. We have to intubate him now.* Then all of a sudden you were just gone.

SONIA: They did one CT scan, and then they did another one because you were deteriorating. They saw something spreading.

> That first CT scan showed two dark spots on my brain: blood seeping through the cracks in my skull and flooding my brainpan. I had suffered a subdural hematoma: a brain hemorrhage that was growing and closing in to kill me. My heart rate had plummeted to forty-four beats per minute.

MEGAN GREENWELL: I signed the paperwork for them to intubate you. It was the least bad option. Their tone was *We're doing this. Somebody sign their name on the paper.*

SAMER KALAF: That's when I realized, *There's a very good chance that Drew may die.* I knew that intubation was normally a thing that you do not come back from.

MEGAN GREENWELL: We still hadn't gotten Sonia's phone number. There was a nice nurse who was like, *You need to find his wife's* *phone number right now. Right this second.* She didn't say because she was afraid you were going to die. But that was the implication.

VICTOR JEFFREYS: When they come back and said there's blood in your brain, it got really scary. I remember getting your bank card and calling them to get your emergency contact number. I'm begging this fucking person at the bank to just call your wife. He wouldn't do it. I was losing it on the phone. I tell Megan, *The hospital has to call the cops.*

MEGAN GREENWELL: I called the police and they said they wouldn't give me your wife's number. And I said, *Well then, will you go to her house?* They said, *You have to have the hospital call.*

At this point, I'd walked outside because it was noisy in the hospital. It was so cold. I'm walking around in a tank top that was under my jacket, just freezing my ass off. I was like, *Can I run back inside and just give them the phone?* They said, *No, they have to call from a hospital line.* So then a nice nurse called immediately.

SONIA: There was a pounding on the door. 2:00 or 3:00 A.M. I heard it and I thought they would go away, but the dog was barking. I came down and looked out the living room window and I saw cop car lights on. I thought it was the police warning me about something in the neighborhood. The cop handed me a note and said, *I'm sorry to tell you this but there's been an accident with your husband in New York. This is all the information we have.* The note was the phone number to the hospital. That's all they told me. I had been dead asleep and completely out of it. So I didn't know what to expect next.

MEGAN GREENWELL: The hospital put me in touch with Sonia. She sounded disoriented and panicked. And extremely worried.

SONIA: They put Megan on the phone and I talked to her for a while. She sounded frazzled but under control. I'd never talked to her before, but I could tell she was scared.

They called me and said they were transferring you by ambulance uptown (to Mount Sinai Hospital) because you needed surgery. They said you fell. They asked if I consented to the surgery. I was like, *Do whatever you need to.* The specifics of the surgery they told me were such a blur.

In the middle of everything going on, here were the kids getting ready for school. I said, *Dad had an accident. He is in a hospital. I'm going to go up to New York. Oma and Opa are coming when you get home from school. I might be gone all weekend, but I'll be back.* I tried to downplay it, and they were fine. They all got off to school. After everyone had left the bus stop, I saw my friend Joel. I said to her, *I gotta tell you something.*

And I burst into tears.

CRANIOTOMY

THE MORNING OF DECEMBER 6

Once Beth Israel radiologists discovered my brain hemorrhage, they realized that I was at the wrong hospital to treat it. Only a certain number of trauma surgeons were on call at that hour in the city. The one I needed, Dr. John Caridi, operated out of Mount Sinai Hospital, which was where Dr. David Heller also happened to practice and was located over eighty blocks away. Back into an ambulance I went. My parents, living eighty miles outside of the city, remained completely unaware of the situation.

MEGAN GREENWELL: Victor and I went in a cab behind the ambulance to Mount Sinai. They told me you had a bleed, but they didn't tell me the context. I have no memory of being in the cab at all.

VICTOR JEFFREYS: I remember walking through that big lobby of Mount Sinai. We're dressed nice. We're walking fast, looking insane.

SAMER KALAF: We had to walk up these stairs, walk to the other side of this building, walk to an elevator. I don't remember the exact path. I just remember there was a lot of walking. And then it was a waiting room with no lighting. I was so exhausted that I fell asleep without even realizing it.

VICTOR JEFFREYS: I remember seeing them wheel you out for surgery. I told somebody else in that room, *That was probably him.* Maybe I'm being crazy. I knew that there was a very, very, very serious possibility that you would die.

MEGAN GREENWELL: Victor and I saw you go by us on the stretcher, in the emergency ward. You looked like a dying person. It was really fucking scary.

DR. JOHN CARIDI (associate professor of neurosurgery, Mount Sinai): I'm trained to do complex spine surgery. But when I'm on call, I take care of all aspects of neurosurgery. Your type of surgery I had probably done, I would say, maybe 150 to 200 times before I did it on you.

VICTOR JEFFREYS: I remember getting home and totally losing it to my roommate. If I slept, it would have been a couple of hours.

MEGAN GREENWELL: I paced around the waiting room for a while. I tried to sleep, but it didn't work. I was all of a sudden alone. That was the worst time. I was definitely afraid you were going to die. I remember being like, *Oh my God, Drew's wife, who has been described to me as an extremely kind person, is going to hate me. How did this happen where, like, I killed Drew?* I was feeling so bad. Sonia was so far away.

SONIA: I called your parents and your mom was like, *Oh, that doesn't sound good. Okay. Good luck.* And hung up. Fast. I think she was just confused and didn't understand the gravity of the situation.

MY MOM: Sonia called us around 3:00 A.M. I was shocked. I said, *Let me get my head together.* I called her right back and said, *We'll get* *in the car.* Then I called Amanda [my sister] and Alex [my brother] and told them that you had a bad accident and we were on our way down, and Amanda just started sobbing. It was terrible. She said, *You have to please come get me.*

I knew it would add time to our trip, but I couldn't refuse. Just sobbing, the poor child.

AMANDA (my sister): Mom called and I thought, *Why is she calling me at four thirty in the morning?* I called her back and she said, *Oh, Drew had just a little accident.* And then I said, *What do you mean, a little accident?* She was like, *Oh, I think he has to have emergency brain surgery, but it's okay. Don't worry, you don't have to come.*

I think she was in shock. I called her back and said, *Emergency brain surgery is not a little accident. You're going to pick me up on your way, and I'll help you drive.* They got here and then it must've taken like five or six hours to get into New York.

MY DAD: By the time we got Amanda, we were beginning to get into rush hour and we just had a terrible wall of traffic as we were going down.

DR. JOHN CARIDI: The hematoma was . . . I don't want to say it was massive, but it was large and in a very precarious spot. Your brain is only 10 percent of your body weight, but gets 25 percent of your blood supply. It has a lot of significant arteries, and those arteries have to drain into the venous system. And so there are what we refer to as venous sinuses. Your hemorrhage was overlying the confluence of the sinuses. It was starting to compress your cerebellum into your brain stem. That can kill you pretty quickly. So while it wasn't the largest hematoma, it was in a very bad spot. If you're not taken to surgery within four hours of that hematoma, then you have no chance of living.

My operation commenced at 6:16 a.m., over six hours after I collapsed.

MOM: Oh my God. It was the worst traffic ever. Your dad got off and tried to do an alternate route, but it was hell.

SONIA: I didn't want to deal with the train station or the airport, so I got on the bus to New York at ten. It was empty. I sat by myself, which was nice. My friend Joel gave me a little goody bag with tissues, some cash, and some snacks. I was telling everybody on the phone what had happened. I had to call work and tell them I wasn't coming. At some point I'd had enough with texting people and I was just playing some music. "Three Little Birds" was the first song. I cried. I take those signs very seriously.

DR. DAVID HELLER: I looked at the CT scans myself using my medical authorization before I went to see you.

MEGAN GREENWELL: David called me. He had seen the scans. He was trying not to say, *I'm not sure he's going to make it,* but it was very clear that he was saying, *I'm not sure he's going to make it.*

DR. DAVID HELLER: I could see the blood on the CT scans. A huge swath of the back of the skull and brain area was filled with blood. Typically, it is very bad when that amount of blood fills that zone. It tends to compress the brain and its vital structures. The position of your brain had shifted. Your midline shift, the central dividing line of the two halves of the brain, was no longer in the center of your skull, and that is super extremely not good. I could not believe that you were going to live at all.

AMANDA: I had a really bad feeling in the car about it. I didn't want to say anything to Mom and Dad. I think it's connected to my own thirteen years of experience working at a children's hospital. Because when kids went to the ICU, that was a bad sign. A high likelihood of being fatal. That's immediately what went in my head.

But I didn't say any of that.

DR. JOHN CARIDI: We flipped you over onto your belly, shaved the back of your head, made a vertical incision down the back, and moved the scalp away. As I recall, there was a linear fracture through that area. So then we used a drill—like a dentist drill, but a little bit more, uh, robust—to make holes in the skull. We connected each one of those holes. Four corners. We connected those corners with a drill that has a foot plate on it, so it wouldn't damage anything underneath.

AMANDA: Mom and Dad refused to let me drive. I kept saying, *I want to drive.* They were driving forty miles an hour where we could have driven sixty. I think they were trying to be calm and get there. I'm like, *You might want to step on it a little bit.*

DAD: I was able to keep it together while driving. I think you get focused on what has to be done and that casts aside other reactions that might otherwise come to the surface.

DR. JOHN CARIDI: We lifted up the bone and there was the rather large hematoma under there. We sucked it out, washed it out, and saw where there was damage to the sinus. And so what you do is you use a small patch of collagen that's mixed with thrombin, which promotes coagulation. That little patch stops that bleeding and seals up that hole in the sinus. Once we made sure that there was no other bleeding, we took the bone and put it back on with tiny plates and screws that fixed the bone in place.

ALEX (my brother): I remember the tone of Mom's voice and how scared and concerned she was, and it was *very* disconcerting.

MOM: It was December 6. Alex's birthday. *Hi, Alex. Happy birthday. Your brother is in dire shape.*

DR. JOHN CARIDI: Because of the location of your hemorrhage, you had a blockage of how your spinal fluid was exiting your brain. Spinal fluid is made in your brain. If it doesn't get out of your brain, it gets backed up and you get what we call hydrocephalus, or water on your brain. That can also be fatal.

ALEX: I was not in the best mental state in the car because I was so worried. But I was very focused on doing the driving to get down there. Did I drive faster than usual? Probably a little bit. I tend to drive pretty fast anyway. Definitely above the speed limit.

DR. JOHN CARIDI: We turned you back over, shaved a small patch on the front of your head, and then inserted a catheter into the fluid-filled part of your brain in order to prevent that accumulation of fluid.

MEGAN GREENWELL: Your family came. It was clear they were yours because they look like you.

AMANDA: Megan met us at the door of the waiting room and explained what had happened. She was obviously upset but clear and focused, trying to explain all the details that she knew. We were all focused on what happened. *How are we in this situation right now?* We were not understanding what happened to you. No one could explain it. *How could he have gone from karaoke singing to being intubated? How the hell does that happen? Did he get beaten up? Did somebody push him? Did something happen that they don't want to tell us?*

MEGAN GREENWELL: I had this defensive instinct because I didn't want them to think it was my fault. But I also hadn't had time to think through whether it *was* my fault. So I was like, *Don't seem defensive. Just tell them what happened.* Your sister was so sweet and she was just crying and crying and crying and crying. Your parents were so nice. *They* were trying to console *me*.

HOWARD: I got to the trauma unit, where people were congregating, and I found Megan and Victor. I was shocked because I had just seen you the night before. I had pictures of you and me from the show. I was showing Megan and other people those pictures. I don't know why I was doing that, but it was like *Drew is fine. He was fine last night*!

MEGAN GREENWELL: It was all so traumatic that exhaustion was not top of mind. The only physical sensation that was really extreme was I had been wearing heels at the event and I didn't have any other shoes. At that point, my feet were numb. They stayed numb for a couple of weeks after that.

They were good shoes, too.

SPINAL DRIP

DECEMBER 6–9

After surgery, doctors at Mount Sinai put me into an induced coma, so that my brain could rest and heal without Awake Drew barging in and fucking everything up. Surgeons had mowed two ski slopes through my hair to make their incisions. I had also busted a blood vessel in my left eye. A red line ran down from the edge of my iris to my lower eyelid and then dashed along the eyelid. Surrounding the eye was a massive shiner, the result of my face smashing into the karaoke bar floor after the back of my head had ricocheted against the wall. I looked *dead*.

AMANDA: Mom and Dad went in first, cause there's only two people at a time. They came out and they were a wreck. I saw you and the first thing that went through my head was that you were going to die.

DAD: I don't remember having big discussions about what your prognosis was. Each of us kept that to ourselves. Your mom and I probably had more emotions about Sonia than anything else. Trying to fathom what she was going through was just unbearable. Just unbearable.

MOM: Your dad and I hugged each other and said, *How do we live in a world without our son?* But that would be about it. It's not my nature to dwell on something like that. And honestly, everybody was busy trying to save you and make sure you were fine. It's just not what's on your mind. Afterward you think, *Oh my God.*

AMANDA: Your head looked like it got peeled open. But I didn't say that to you. I didn't want to freak you out. You had the spinal fluid drip, which needed to stay level with your head. Otherwise the pressure in your head would kill you.

DR. DAVID HELLER: They were monitoring it like a tire gauge. It's this thing called intracranial pressure. The blood doesn't kill you because you bleed to death, but because it compresses the brain. So they put in a probe that runs through a hole in your skull, and they have it running up to a machine 24/7 to keep your intracranial pressure within one level or another. You looked about as sick as anybody looks.

AMANDA: I didn't know that they were sedating you. I thought that you were actually not waking up.

DAD: When we first saw you, you were really in much more terrible shape than we could have imagined. I had to spend an awful lot of time holding your hand and saying, *Can you feel mine?* I was getting no reaction at all other than your breathing. Your breathing.

AMANDA: Having no response when I squeezed your hand was really frightening because it showed you were not doing well.

ALEX: Just seeing you in person that first time after the accident was jarring. It really drives it home that this is real and happening. You looked so helpless. Not moving or anything.

HOWARD: It was a long wait to see you. When I saw you, I got really upset and I started to break down. You looked horrible. I mean really, really bad.

AMANDA: Howard came in with all these Dunkin' Donuts Munchkins and coffee. I'm like, *I'm gonna throw up. I can't even imagine eating. I don't want a fucking Munchkin with jelly, I'm about to vomit all over the place as it is.* But it was really nice.

Then Howard went in to see you and he was really shaken up. He was obviously crying when he came out.

HOWARD: Your eyes were swollen and purple. Parts of your head were exposed, were partially shaved. You had a breathing tube. You were pissing into a bag. You could see all the inner workings, all the tubes: two coming out of your head, draining fluid into a bag. I'm sorry. I'm actually getting a little bit choked up right now.

JESSE: There was still blood in your hair and scalp. You had a big cut in the front of your head and your eyes were black.

AMANDA: I had your bag and they wanted me to get your car keys so Sonia's dad could find your car, because it was parked in a DC garage.

It was horrible, looking through your stuff. It was like you had died. That really stuck with me. Then I saw your contact lens case. I'm like, *Oh my God, they're still in his eyes.* They took your contacts out and then I got your glasses.

HOWARD: I'd like to say that I had faith that you were gonna be okay, but I didn't. After seeing you, it was hard to imagine a world in which you were going to recover fully.

AMANDA: The first time I went in and came back, I lost it in the waiting room. I don't know how to explain it. It's impossible to control how you're feeling. I remember people in the waiting room looking at us and I could tell they were like, *Oh, here we go again.*

> At one point during my coma, I aspirated: throwing up while lying in bed and then breathing the vomit back in, triggering respiratory failure. They hooked me up to a ventilator, a machine that would soon prove both invaluable and scarce in New York during the initial stages of the coronavirus pandemic. When they took me off the ventilator, I aspirated again. Back on I went. Dad says the doctors had to go into my lungs with microscopic tweezers to remove bits of solid regurgitate.

HOWARD: You smelled rank. As the days would go by, the smell got even worse.

JESSE: Your smell was not good. It was the odor of a man who'd been sitting in his own filth for a while.

SONIA: They had to clean you, since you were not getting up to use the bathroom. You smelled like sterile hospital: dried alcohol and dirty hair.

FLORA (my daughter): [Gives thumbs-down and holds her nose when she overhears me asking Sonia how I smelled in the hospital.]

HOWARD: You weren't shaving, obviously. You have very unappealing face stubble, so that didn't help your look either.

DAD: I was operating under the assumption that you weren't even fifty-fifty to live. I think I was operating under the assumption that this might be it.

AMANDA: I remember thinking what I would do when you died. How I would help Sonia. I could move down there for a while. I could do all these different things.

BARRY PETCHESKY: You looked so small. So withered and diminished physically. Completely unconscious.

AMANDA: Byrd came into the hospital, looking like he was like right off the runway with his tweed suit. I'm like, *Oh my God, who is this person?*

BYRD LEAVELL (friend, also my book agent): Your family was there in that waiting room. It couldn't have been heavier. Everyone looked like they got hit in the stomach with a baseball bat. Just thousand-yard stares. I was already scared, and then I saw them and I got *really* scared.

Seeing you . . . It just didn't look like something that anyone would ever recover from.

AMANDA: He and I were in there and tearing up and then he was talking to you like, *Fuck you. You have to wake up, dude.* That was helpful because, for me, it was like he was talking to a normal person instead of this fragile person who's going to die. It was really funny. Thank God.

BYRD LEAVELL: I thought I was saying goodbye to you, but also I was trying to get into your head to say something positive.

AMANDA: They later explained to us that the hematoma was pressing on your brain stem, which was the cause of many deaths that I'd seen in the ICU. I was worried that maybe there was no brain activity. Like, brain death already.

BYRD LEAVELL: I was trying to be of service in any possible way to a family that was in it together and was clearly still processing how something like this could happen. We were all like, *Did Drew do this to himself by being an idiot?*

I walked out of Mount Sinai crying.

AMANDA: They started testing your reflexes to see if you were responding, and you weren't, which is what was scaring me. They were bringing your sedation down and you weren't doing much at all. I got freaked out because they warned us that you could be in a nursing home for the rest of your life with severe brain damage.

SONIA: Amanda and Susie Banikarim met me outside Mount Sinai. Amanda's always got her heart on her face. She looked very concerned and confused. They told me you were sedated, and I didn't really understand what that meant.

Your parents looked tired and scared. Your mom had big tears in her eyes.

MEGAN GREENWELL: Your sister asked a bunch of good questions. They were definitely in investigation mode. I went through the process of explaining what had happened. And then she politely said, *Okay, why don't you leave it to the family now?*

SONIA: I was pissed at Deadspin. I didn't know what they put you through the day [of the awards], and I knew you weren't feeling well. I felt like they owed me. So I said to Susie, *Send me a car.* She paid the driver extra to have him wait outside Port Authority, which was nice.

SUSIE BANIKARIM (Gizmodo Media Group executive editor): My impression of Sonia through the whole thing was that she was just a very no-nonsense person.

DR. DAVID HELLER: I remember Sonia being very calm and very poised, but with tears in her eyes. And she was definitely trying to focus on being composed in that way.

BYRD LEAVELL: The first time I was there, Sonia went in by herself. She came out and she'd been crying. That was the only time I saw her cry. She had clearly had her moment with you.

DR. DAVID HELLER: I explained to Sonia, *This number here on this screen, we want it to be between here and here. Here's his breathing rate, his blood pressure. All these numbers are good.* And it was gratifying to tell Sonia that, because what you looked like *didn't* reflect it.

SONIA: I may have had a veneer of normalcy, but inside I was a hot mess. I called my doctor that Monday morning and I said, *I need an appointment for drugs.* They could tell over the phone. Dr. Corden was like, *Girl, you need some Xanax, you need some Ambien.*

Xanax took the edge off right away. Before that, I was shaking. I was nauseous. I had no appetite, nothing. My friend Kristin brought me that Cup of Calm tea. That's the only thing I could drink.

BARRY PETCHESKY: Sonia was totally quiet. She wouldn't take her eyes off you.

DR. JOHN CARIDI: I remember meeting Sonia in the ICU and telling her that I felt pretty strongly that you were going to be okay. That it was going to be a bumpy road, but that ultimately you would do well. You were going to need a lot of rehab. She looked shockingly calm. Asked a lot of pointed and appropriate questions. She wasn't hysterical or anything like that. She was very in control. [Laughs.] Probably not like my wife would be.

I was confident, given your injury, that you were going to recover. But it's always difficult to say what *percentage* you're going to recover.

HOWARD: When you first came out of surgery, your neurosurgeon came out. He gave a not-very-uplifting assessment. He was circumspect and ambiguous. He's like, *We won't know for a couple of days, but it's certainly not without possibility that he's not the person that you remember.* I was shocked. I didn't believe it. It was devastating to hear, almost impossible for me to get my head around. I was still ruminating on the fact that I had seen you just the evening before.

SONIA: Amanda and I were constantly hugging and crying with each other. She was so supportive. I couldn't have gone through it with anybody else. Honestly. I know it.

PATRICK REDFORD (writer, Deadspin): Minutes after I arrived at the office the next morning, Megan asked me to return to the hotel to pack your room up. Waves of dread passed over me as I became aware that the spectrum of possibilities included death.

The hotel staff let me into your room, where I learned what a garment bag was as I tried to fold up your stuff. It must have been the mundanity of folding clothes or trying to organize your Dopp kit, but at some point, I could not stop thinking, *This is someone's dad. There are three kids who rely on Drew. He can't die.*

BARRY PETCHESKY: I'm a pretty positive person. So most of the time I felt like, *He's gotten what he needed. This is a really good hospital with really good doctors. This is one of the best, like, brain hospitals in the country. He's going to be okay.* And then there were times I would start questioning it. *What if he's not? What if I never see Drew alive again? What if he dies?* I refused to let myself spend time with those thoughts.

ALEX: I wanted you to wake up so that I could talk to you and get a sense of *Where are you?*

DAD: There was this nagging desire to see if we can get some sort of a physical reaction out of you, because then that would mean that you were actually alive instead of just *theoretically* alive. We would tap your hand and then say, *Tap back if you can hear.* Every now and then, you would. But you weren't coming to or anything like that.

ALEX: We were holding your hand, touching your shoulder . . . letting you know that we were there. *Hi, Drew. It's Alex. It's Mom. It's whoever. We're here with you. We love you so much and really want you to get better.* That you were squeezing let us know that *you* knew we were there. Or at least that's what I hoped it meant.

MOM: Alex was so dear. He would pat you on the chest and say, *Come on, buddy, come on.* Oh God.

JESSE: There were moments where it seemed like you could hear what was going on.

ERICA (friend, Howard's sister): I was really scared. I was worried about losing you, and I kept wanting to know the odds. I read about other brain conditions. *Are there people recovering from this? And if you are able to wake up and recover, what kind of life can you have?* Obviously nobody can answer that, because nobody knows how anybody is going to come out of that, because the brain is such a sensitive organ.

SONIA: You looked like shit. You did not look like you. It was like when Colin was in the NICU: a whole bunch of tubes and machines. You know they're helping, but you don't know what they do. Like an alien hooked up. You were completely out of it.

You reacted when I came in. Maybe a little tear. All the machines were constantly beeping. I said to you, *What did you do? Shithead. You better come back. You owe me.*

HOWARD: Your dad's much less emotional than your mom, but there were times where he would turn bright pink and was super upset. He was very tender. He kept calling you "buddy," too. *Come on, buddy.*

AMANDA: I said, *Hi, Drew. It's Amanda. You look like shit.* I was trying to be funny because I wanted to make light of it. Mom was with me and I was trying to be calm for her, because she was not doing very well. Sometimes you would have a tear on your eye. I don't know if you were crying.

HOWARD: The doctors said it was important for people that you knew to talk to you to make those synaptic connections. I remember telling you what happened. I remember holding your hand and telling you that I was here. *You're gonna be okay.*

JESSE: I asked you if you wanted to hear some music. I played you some Queens of the Stone Age at one point. Juri (Howard's cousin) was there a bunch. He had reached out to a Buddhist temple in Nepal to pray for you.

AMANDA: You were never alone. Alex was there a lot, and Alex was incredibly sweet, holding your hand and talking softly. That always made me cry. Alex was tearing up most of the time when he was in there.

HOWARD: Sometimes if your family was leaving, they'd ask me to stay a little longer, so I helped fill the gaps to make sure you weren't alone.

JESSE: When you were comatose, they would open your eyes to look at them. You were totally checked out. In another place. So it was tough seeing you like that.

HOWARD: I remember your mom breaking down crying and me hugging her. She was saying, *Drew's got this marvelous, marvelous mind.* She was holding your hand, stroking your hair. Your mom would tell me it was so important you know you're not by yourself.

AMANDA: You would squeeze my hand a little, but it was hard to tell if it was just a random movement or not. You started squeezing Sonia's hand more and more.

ALEX: We were really worried whether or not you would be you after all of this. Would you be able to drive a car? Would you be able to work? Could you cook? Could you walk around the house without help? We had no idea and that was very, very scary. For a long time it seemed like odds were against it.

AMANDA: We met with the surgeon, Dr. Caridi. He kept saying, *The next couple of days are the critical time. It's going to go one way or the other.* There were so many other ways that things could go wrong. There was no hope given at all. No one said anything about you surviving. That was what scared me.

DR. DAVID HELLER: Dr. Caridi was courteous and kind, but for the first few seconds I was dreadfully afraid that he was going to say that you would die, because frankly, that's what I thought was the most likely scenario, based on what I saw in the CT scans.

DAD: At one point we had a discussion with David Heller. I remember trying to build a story out of the tone of voice he was using, to figure out how serious this really was. It bothered me that I didn't hear as many platitudes as I wanted to hear. We got a few clues that this was really serious shit.

MOM: The main thing that got us at the beginning was *Oh my God, he had brain surgery.* It's not like heart surgery or anything else. Brain surgery is a whole other thing.

DR. DAVID HELLER: Dr. Rothrock [the neurosurgery resident] showed us two scans. The "before" was the same one that I looked at where I was like, *Good God, that's very bad.* Then he said, *We were able to fix it and now it looks like this.* I was like, *Oh my God.* I couldn't believe it. You didn't even need medical training to see the difference. I was like, *These are the same brain?* It was really fucking dramatic.

Dr. Rothrock said, *Drew is not going to die today of this. On the other hand, he is going to have an extraordinarily long recovery. This is a whole new era in this human being's life. This is going to take months. Maybe years. It remains to be seen how long it's going to take, if ever, for him to get back to normal, and it's never going to be the same normal for this person.*

SONIA: I was being buried under an avalanche of hot rocks. Hard to breathe. I was just putting one foot in front of the other. That's the only way I could do it.

AMANDA: Every two seconds Alex kept offering me a fricking Twizzler or a bag of M&M's. He ate nonstop crap, like, for three days. I knew he was stressed if he was doing that, because Alex is not like that. I was too upset to eat, because in my mind, like, you were dying. You were going to be dead. I was planning how I would help, like, your kids and Mom and Dad, because I thought that you were not going to survive.

ALEX: I've actually noticed this recently: My way of dealing with stress is actually to eat *more,* not less. So when it was time to go to dinner, I was very ready to eat. I probably ate quite a lot.

MOM: They kicked us out of the hospital from about 5:30 P.M. to 7:00. They had a change of shift, so we left, and there were a couple of nice neighborhood restaurants. It was an Italian place that was particularly comfortable, and we went there. We went out for dinner. I was able to drink.

ALEX: In some ways I remember things outside the hospital better because they were little tiny patches of, I don't know if "fun" is the right word, but little moments where we were not so focused on the negative aspects of what was going on. A break from the trauma of the whole thing.

HOWARD: Your dad ordered a couple of bottles of red wine.

DAD: I was able to drink. I don't think ordinarily I suffer from loss of appetite when I'm upset. Maybe the opposite.

MOM: I don't know that I had the biggest appetite, and I don't love Italian food [note: What the fuck, Mom], but I know I was putting the wine down.

SONIA: That was a beautiful restaurant. What did I eat? I don't know. I excused myself and I went to the bathroom and had a good cry, then came back and it was better. Everybody looked spent.

AMANDA: That was surreal. We were sitting at some restaurant and, like, *Oh my God, what the hell? I cannot pretend that life is normal here.* I may have had a beer.

ALEX: Everybody was trying to function normally, but we weren't, because it wasn't a normal situation at all.

HOWARD: I remember watching a Vikings game with you in the ICU. Your brother was there. We were trying to talk to you about the Vikings game, making sure that game was on for you and, like, talking about the game even though you were unconscious.

JESSE: I went to the hospital and hung out with your folks. I remember I stopped by an Italian pastry shop. I bought a box of cookies, just to have nibbles for them. Your parents were remarkably calm. I sent Howard a text: "These Magarys are tough." And Howard said, "My family would be a disaster." And I'm like, "As would mine."

THE VIGIL

DECEMBER 9 ONWARD

had survived the craniotomy. Now I had to get up. One thing I didn't know before my own coma is that an induced coma is not a consistent one. Doctors periodically bring you out of the coma to see if you're ready and able to start living again.

I was not ready yet. Perhaps I never would be.

AMANDA: It was the nastiest waiting room I've ever been in. Red pleather couches. This one woman took over the couch area because her husband had been there for weeks. Her phone kept going off and the ringtone was a voice saying *RING, RING, RING, RING, RING, RING, RING* over and over again, progressively louder. I'm like, *Oh my God, I'm going to fucking kill her.*

JESSE: She had a really annoying phone ring. It kept going off and she's loudly chatting on the phone. You can't really tell somebody to turn it down a little bit in that situation.

MOM: There were other families in the waiting room. We were all very respectful of one another and quiet. After a while we started to smile and share a few stories. You'd always come in and say, *How's your patient today?* That kind of thing. The other stories were often worse than ours.

SONIA: This is the ICU. This is a high-stress situation. People dying all over the place. The waiting room was the most depressing thing you could imagine. Super dark. Kept cold on purpose. There was a woman in there whose husband had been there for weeks. Lived on the couch and would go into the bathroom and smoke. I was like, *That's disgusting. Can you stop? Everyone needs that bathroom. If you're smoking, go outside. I don't want to smell that.* She was like, *All right. I'm sorry.*

One thing I learned was to speak up for whatever I needed. With complete strangers. I didn't give one shit.

DR. JOHN CARIDI: The people who have a hematoma like this, who get surgery on time, actually do very well. So it all depends on if you're taken to the right place.

ERICA: It was a really disgusting hospital floor, by the way. I remember distinctly being like, *How the fuck is this sterile? How is this the brain trauma area?*

MOM: Neither Sonia nor I slept for a month. Your dear wife was so brave. I don't know how she got through it at the beginning. She said to me, *I'm so scared.* I tried to hold her and comfort her, but she was just a wreck. But she carried on.

ERICA: Sonia was as poised as I could possibly imagine. She was able even to tell me a joke, which I thought was kind of shocking but also made me feel comforted. She was telling me how you were flashing everybody. Showing your twig and berries. She got a giggle out of that.

HOWARD: There were a few times your balls would be hanging out. Your mom was like, *Andrew, can you keep that covered?*

BYRD LEAVELL: Your mom kept calling you Andrew, which was so funny to me.

JESSE: Sometimes you'd shift and your dong would flop out. We were like, *All right, let's cover Drew up, make sure nobody's looking at his balls.*

HOWARD: And then she'd comment: *He keeps trying to show his assets!* She was trying to make light of it. It was funny.

JESSE: I brought some clementines, because I had learned my lesson about bringing cookies. Your folks were so polite and so WASPy and said, *These clementines are just the best.* Like they were at a picnic instead of being stuck in this horrible waiting room while their son was teetering on the brink.

SONIA: Byrd saw your mom walk out of your room, her hair still perfectly coiffed, and said, "That's the stuff of legends."

ERICA: Your mom was on your left. Your dad was on your right and basically didn't leave the entire time I was there. Your dad kept trying to talk to you. You were really agitated. One of your feet was really hot.

HOWARD: As you probably have heard, you were a very restless patient.

ERICA: You were covered in machines.

DAD: Left to your own devices, you'd remove things. You were trying to get rid of things that were bothering you. And violently.

SONIA: One of the doctors told me that your behavior was similar to symptoms of alcohol withdrawal.

HOWARD: Your mom would be trying to restrain you. I remember a few times her coming out of your room and being like, *Howard, can you come help?* You weren't that strong, but you were forceful and you were very wiggly. You were hard to contain.

Your dad would be very upset when he saw you struggling against the restraints. Your dad's a big guy. He's also older. So it was hard seeing your father trying to help restrain you. I think your parents were trying to impress upon you how much effort was being put into getting you through this. Like, *Drew, God, let these people help you.* They were frustrated.

SONIA: They would lessen the sedation to see how you did. You were violent and you pulled your intubation out, which is not good. You were physical and you're a big guy. Some of these nurses are half your size, and it would take two people to come in and hold you down. I can't remember if you were ever strapped down or not, but you probably should have been. They had to hire a nurse to sit with you twenty-four hours to monitor you, which continued all through your stay. I don't know if you know that. [Note: I did not.]

I cornered Susie Banikarim in the hospital hallway and told her we needed a hotel room for a couple of days. I said, *I need to move my family up here. I need an apartment.*

DAD: The Viceroy, where we stayed first, had just been through one of the most devastating sales in the history of the hotel business in New York. I just learned this last night: The hotel had been bought for $150 million. And was being sold for twenty-five. (Note: The actual sale price was $41 million.) I mean, just astounding.

But we enjoyed it.

AMANDA: Sonia and I shared a hotel room. I don't think we slept at all. There was one night we took melatonin. I had an adverse reaction. We were both up all night because of it.

SONIA: Amanda's a great roommate. We shared a bed. I couldn't fall asleep the first night. So at some point I got up to find a piece of paper to write down a list of stuff I had to take care of: what insurance was gonna cover, etc.

MOM: Sonia was on the phone all day long, talking to the insurance people, setting up physical therapy for you at home, neurological visits and everything. Ordinarily the hospital would do this. But because you lived in a different state, they didn't have the connection. She had to do everything herself. At that point she was really, if you don't mind my saying, pretty stressed about finances. She was really having to work hard.

SONIA: I believed in my heart that you would live. I *needed* you to be alive. Your death was not an option. But it was in the back of my mind. I knew we didn't have a will. I knew you were the main earner. After all the hospital stuff, I was like, *We're going to have to sell that house. Live somewhere cheaper.*

ERICA: For my second visit, I asked Sonia what I could bring. She insisted on nothing. I made her baked ziti, just because I wanted her to have something that was homemade.

SUSIE BANIKARIM: To my bosses, I was like, *We're going to do whatever the fuck it takes to take care of this family, and that's not open for discussion.* I didn't give a fuck. I'm like, *Just do it,* you know? And we sorted it. I found an option.

Your family ended up being happy with the apartment. I was very anxious about that, because I found it on Airbnb and you never know. The worst-case scenario is they show up and it's some shithole.

SONIA: It was a great apartment. A fourth-floor walk-up. Your parents hoofed that walk-up twice a day. With groceries.

MOM: It almost killed me. But it kept me in shape.

SONIA: The kids were kind of excited when they came up to New York. Your parents were going to be there. It was an adventure. It was something different.

Years before my accident, I took Rudy and Flora to New York for a couple of nights on my own. We stayed in an Airbnb on the Lower East Side: the kind of Airbnb that its owner clearly lived in for the bulk of the year. Her fridge and her cabinets were still full of leftovers and iced tea and beer, and I had to remind both Flora and Rudy constantly to not touch any of those things. I also had the honor of showing them how window-unit air conditioners worked. Or, more accurately, how they did not.

Our Airbnb for that trip was located on the fifth floor of a fifth-floor walk-up. My kids had never been in a walk-up before. They bitched with every single step up that first climb. But the complaints subsided the following day, and even more the day after that. The cool thing about New York is that anyone gets to feel like they're a New Yorker after living there for just a bit. My kids rewired themselves to be New Yorkers on that trip. They got in rhythm with the city. How it lived. How it moved. After we got back home, I promised Rudy and Flora that we'd make the trip again one day.

AMANDA: We went right to the hospital with the kids. I had taken all these pictures of your room and the machines. I showed the kids that, because I know that that's really helpful preparation for what that looks like.

MOM: Amanda was just magnificent, especially the way she prepped your kids. They didn't seem to be scared at all.

SONIA: The kids were surprised when they saw you. They came over and they hugged you. They didn't want to stay long. Nobody wants to be in a hospital, and they probably got vibes that it was not a good place to be. It was a very serious unit, of course. So they said hi and goodbye. Flora probably stayed the longest. I think the boys got spooked and booked it.

MOM: They were long days. It was a vigil.

AMANDA: I remember bargaining with God. *I'll do anything if you let him live. Whatever it takes. I'll trade myself. I don't care. You can't take him.* I was angry. It wasn't *Oh please, God, in our time of need.* I was pissed. But crap! [Laughs.] Now I have to pay up!

ERICA: I went back to the waiting room and your mom, in Mrs. Magary classic form, was very poised. Your dad was also very calm, which is *so* not Jewish. I found that to be disconcerting, like, *Why isn't there more hysteria?* I knew that that wouldn't help anything, but I just was expecting everybody in your face, like, very Jewish. [Note: Erica is Jewish.]

AMANDA: I went back to work, and when I arrived, we had an emergency right away where I had to take a student to the hospital. I sat there all night with her in the ER, like, *Oh God, I can't handle this.* It took everything out of me to just do that one night.

SONIA: The kids loved the apartment. I mean, they complained about the walk-up, but I let them do whatever they wanted. You want to do iPad? Go for it. I think we rented *Home Alone* a couple of times.

MOM: They had a favorite place on Madison Avenue by the hospital. A little diner. The guy who owned it, a Greek guy, would say, "The usual table?" Then they'd put us in this booth in the back. It was good, fresh food. Rudy was hilarious because he kept saying, *I love this place, Gammy. The service is excellent.* Because the food would come out in about five seconds.

The kids discovered other favorite haunts during their stay. They loved the pizza at a nearby slice chain called

Little Italy, "Little Italy" presumably ranking second to "Ray's" among New York slice joint names. They loved the fries at Parm. Rudy kept fry rankings in his head at all times. Whenever I asked him where a new place's fries ranked, he scrunched up his face and let loose a number within ten seconds. Parm was a top-five fry emporium for him.

On a different venture out, Flora tried fries and gravy for the first time at the Midnight Express diner—a place Sonia used to swear by when we lived in the city and she was dead drunk at 2:00 A.M.—and they were a revelation to her. The kids loved taking taxis everywhere like fancy city people. They probably asked Santa to buy them a loft in Tribeca for this Christmas.

SONIA: Your parents would plan things for the kids every day. Of course, the kids wanted different things, but they made it work. Your dad went to go see *Into the Spider-Verse* with Colin. And he was like, *I have no idea what I just saw.*

MOM: Then we would go to a playground. Our goal was to hit every playground in Central Park, which we just about did. The kids were troopers. We made them walk everywhere. Colin would jump out in the street and say, *TAXI!* and put his hand up. I'd say, *No, Colin, not yet. No, no. You got five more blocks.*

SONIA: I would take the kids on the bus just so they wouldn't get spoiled taking cabs everywhere.

MOM: We tried to keep them outside and keep them running. They couldn't stay in the hospital for a long time. It was pretty dreary.

SONIA: I downplayed it with the kids. I said, *He's being taken care of. He's going to be okay.* They were worried, but they got it and kept on going. I remembered that it's always good to keep them on a schedule and keep them occupied. One of the boys or both of them were sick when we first got there. That was fun. Colin was watching TV all the time the first weekend. I was sitting there like, *What am I going to do?* I was sad and scared and I told them that, but I also didn't want to seem like it was the end of the world. I mean, it *would* have been the end of the world if you hadn't made it.

MOM: The other good thing that came out of it was we really had a wonderful bonding experience with your kids because, yes, we all get together and we love each other and blah, blah, blah. But we'd never really *lived* with them before. The fact that we were with them so many hours a day, it was wonderful. We loved that.

AMANDA: The apartment was like you're in a normal New York mode of *Hey, I'm just coming home.* But *Oh, because Drew is in the hospital.*

SONIA: Your parents had moved into the apartment the day before we did. They brought their stuff, plus groceries and a full bar. There was a bar cart in the dining room. When I got there, it was completely stocked. A month later, empty. They quit drinking later on, but they went out with a bang.

AMANDA: Sonia and I walked up to the hospital together every day. It must've been forty blocks. Then we just sat in the hospital all day, taking turns being with you whenever we could. We told the staff a lot about you so that they would know you as a person.

MOM: We got into a nice rhythm with the kids. Because we always wanted to cover you, your dad and I would get up, have coffee, and go to the hospital early. Sonia and the kids would sleep and chill in the morning, then get up to the hospital around noon. Then we would babysit. That was our job.

AMANDA: Mom was texting me at like five in the morning, like, *I'm going to walk to the hospital. I know I can't get in, but I'm just gonna go sit there.*

SONIA: Your parents, you know, they get up at the crack of ass. I didn't want to rush the kids out the door, because they were rushed out all the time for school. So we would sleep. I needed to sleep. I hit up your mom for an Ambien, actually. I was like, *You got some of that stuff? Will you share?* And she was like, *All right.*

DAD: The days were all very similar. Which day was which I could never figure out. Our whole focus was being at your bedside.

SONIA: I would call every morning for an update, then again before lunch, usually eleven o'clock. Your parents would take the kids to lunch at the diner and I would stay with you for the rest of the day. Then we would switch back.

I would sit in your room for six hours. I could never tell if they were trying to get the bed empty and move you on, or if you really were ready to go to the next stage of recovery. They had to do everything gradually. They would lessen the sedation to see how you reacted. And then, to feed you, you had a tube. I haven't thought about any of this stuff in a long time. I apologize. I don't remember a lot of these details.

AMANDA: They took your sedation down further, and the nurse came in and said, *If you can hear me, like, put up two fingers.* You flipped them off, and we started crying and laughing. The nurse was like, *That's the happiest I've ever been being flipped off in my life.* That to me was when things shifted.

SONIA: The nurse came in to lessen your sedation again. It was time to test you. She said, *Can you show me two fingers?* And you gave everyone the double bird with your eyes still closed. We all laughed and cried. The nurse was like, *All right, that works.*

MOM: The nurse came in and she was shouting at you, *DREW, DREW, CAN YOU HEAR ME?* She said, *Give me a finger.* Then you gave her *the* finger. So we all said, *Oh, he's okay.* That was the milestone, all right.

ALEX: We still hadn't had a lot of indications that you were still yourself. That was one of the first.

MEGAN GREENWELL: When you gave that nurse the double bird, we heard about that pretty immediately.

MOM: I leaned in to you, and you kept kissing my face like a baby or a doggy would do. Do you know what I mean? I would say, *It's Mom. It's Mom.* And it tore my heart out. It was heartwarming. The fact that there was a sign of life there was a miracle.

AN INVESTIGATION

I was thirsty, so thirsty I thought I was gonna swallow my own throat. Despite waking up and knowing who I was, I was still loopy from all of the terrifying, fantastic coma drugs. When you're in a hospital, you get to legally enjoy the effects of fentanyl. You *have* to take it. It's a win-win for everyone involved. But as a result of that medically necessary high, I came back into the world somewhat . . . delusional. How delusional? Well now, lemme take you on a tour through my varying states of altered consciousness.

First of all, I believed the entire hospital was on rails, and that it shuttled regularly between New York, Boston, and Los Angeles. At one point Dad came to visit and I was like, *Oh wow, you flew all the way to LA just to see me!* And he was like, *Drew, what are you talking about? We're in New York.* And I was like, *SURE, OLD MAN. NICE TRY. I DON'T THINK SO.*

I also believed, for some reason, that a celebrity chef (no idea who) was killed at the same karaoke bar the night when I bashed my skull in, and that *I* was a person of interest in that chef's death. Please know that no famous chef died that night, nor have I ever murdered anyone. At least, not that you know of. The fentanyl was telling me that the chef worked at the Chateau Marmont hotel in LA and that my rolling hospital was connected to the Chateau whenever it was stationed there. It made me very nervous. At any second, I expected a plainclothes detective to come in and grill me into fessing up.

Simultaneously, I believed that everyone *else* in the hospital believed that I was a Mexican special forces officer, and that they were all making a concerted effort to get me back on duty and preserve my cover. One night I had to shit into a bedpan, and I imagined all the nurses and techs taking my stool sample to a lab for extensive study, making sure it was still consistent with the indigenous peoples of Chiapas. *Oh wow, it's an exact match! This guy . . . this guy is good.*

Another time, when the staff wheeled me on a gurney down to a lower level for a CT scan, I found myself under another delusion: that I was being taken into an audition for *Suicide Squad 2*. For my imagined Suicide Squequel, I thought that the studio had made the executive decision to merge the DC cinematic universe with the Harry Potter cinematic universe. Hence, my character would be a new addition to the bad-guy squad but *also* a Hogwarts train proctor. No such movie exists.

I also thought the catheter tube inside me had a thin brown roll, the consistency of a dog biscuit, running through it and into my penis. I tried, unsuccessfully, to yank the whole apparatus out. Do NOT attempt such a thing. As I fought my way out of the fog, I had little ability to discern between the real and the fantastical. I needed lucidity, and I needed the truth. Sonia was already working to uncover the latter.

JESSE: They would bring you out of sedation, and you would immediately come back to whatever semblance of yourself you were at that point and want to shift because you were in agony. Also you had this fucking tube in your throat. Your dad and I had to prevent you from ripping the thing out. You were not a happy camper when you were awake.

AMANDA: Did Sonia tell you about when the psychiatrist—a person came to evaluate you for the rehab unit? When they asked you about who's the president of the United States, you went on and on. *That fucking piece of shit*, blah, blah blah. Then the doctor came around the curtain. She was like, *Well, sometimes people can be a little bit agitated or, like, say things they don't mean when they've had a head injury.* I'm like, *Oh, no, no, no. Actually, that is pretty accurate.*

MATT UFFORD: You looked awful. You were exhausted by everything immediately. Being awake was a big wear on you. You would get into Frankenstein's-monster mode and couldn't voice your feelings beyond *I'm thirsty.*

AMANDA: Mom worked really hard to be with the kids while Sonia would visit you.

SONIA: Honestly, you were kind of a jackass. You didn't want to sit up. You withdrew. You were never super chatty. I would talk to you and you'd be happy for a little bit. And then you would settle in and be quiet. And I would leave it.

HOWARD: You kept on telling me you were in so much pain because of your back. You were begging them to flatten the bed out.

SONIA: I got to know the nurses and asked them a zillion questions. *What's that? What does that do? Why is that number like that? Can you take him off of that?* You looked very uncomfortable. I kept telling every new nurse, *He's got a bad back. He's going to be complaining about this.* You had a drain that had to be at a certain angle. So they worked with me and we put you halfway. You could not be completely flat.

AMANDA: I started despising New York. I felt like it represented the worst thing that had ever happened in my life. I remember going to Dunkin' Donuts, getting some coffee, and then always looking around at people. *They're fine and they have no idea what's* *going on in my head.* It would make me angry that they got to go on with their normal lives.

I refused to go back to New York for a long time. And then we went back with my son to get his special shoes at the Nike store when they came out on his birthday [in December 2019]. That was a really great day. That created some new memories. I have all these other awful, horrible memories.

SONIA: I talked to Byrd. Not so much about lawsuits, but just wrongful harm. He gave me good advice. He was like, *Be very careful with them. They're pretty slick.* Not Susie and Megan. They were human. But when it came time to deal with the Univision people that I got in touch with [Note: Univision owned Deadspin at the time], he was like, *Just be careful. Be on guard.*

I told Megan I would like to get together with everybody who was there and find out what really happened.

MEGAN GREENWELL: Sonia asked me, Victor, Jorge, and Susie to come to the hospital to interview us about what had happened, step by step. So we did that in the cafeteria at Sinai.

JORGE CORONA: Sonia and your dad were looking for answers. Sonia had a pad in front of her, trying to piece together everything that happened.

SONIA: Everybody was scared. Kind of cautious. I don't know what kind of vibe I gave off. I told them I just wanted to get the information. I'm like, *I'm not looking to go after you. I'm not going to sue you. I just want to know what happened that night.*

MEGAN GREENWELL: She asked us everything. It took a couple of hours. I was a little nervous about it going in. I didn't know if Sonia wanted to hold us responsible. But it was very straightforward. It was clear that they were on a fact-finding mission, and we didn't leave anything out for them. It didn't feel tense to me.

SUSIE BANIKARIM: But it definitely didn't feel chill, either. At that point, we still really didn't know if you were going to recover. We said, *Here's the information. It is the best information we have, but we know it doesn't make sense, and we don't know how to answer that part of it.*

DR. DAVID HELLER: Your blood alcohol level that night was 16.2 milligrams per deciliter, which corresponds to a BAL of 0.0162. Basically the level you'd get to after 0.5 to 1 beer. Your tox screen was done at 2:22 A.M. It's possible you had two drinks' worth in your system when you had collapsed hours earlier. Marijuana screen was negative. As was, for what it's worth, cocaine, methadone, opiates, and PCP.

JORGE CORONA: Your dad was very quiet. He wasn't asking too many questions. Sonia was asking the most questions. They were both wonderful and thankful. Sonia gave us hugs. I think we shook hands with your dad.

VICTOR JEFFREYS: Your wife and father asked us to recount our story. You hear me recounting it now. Imagine it for your wife.

> After the sit-down, my parents decided to return to the scene of the crime, if there actually had been one.

DAD: I kind of coerced your mother into going to the karaoke bar because I said, *We are never ever, ever gonna be able to see this again, and we better have some understanding about what really happened.*

It was a strange visit, because the people who were representing the management let your mom and me go around and look at anything we wanted. They weren't standing guard over us, which surprised me. There was no defensiveness on their part. If they were, they were under perfect instructions to say nothing. We went around and looked at everything that we possibly could. There's nothing dingier than a place like that during the daytime. I'm glad there wasn't a fire there, because you all would have died in the fire.

HOWARD: They said that they found you splayed on the ground next to a credenza or something in this narrow hallway?

MEGAN GREENWELL: No, no, there was nothing in the hallway.

DR. DAVID HELLER (after I asked him if I could have suffered a brain bleed and then, in a fit of mania, intentionally driven my head into the wall): These kinds of hemorrhages, although they will obviously make you altered mentally, will not alter you in a way that will make you do spontaneous, violent, dis-inhibited things. You become less aware of who you are as different parts of your brain start to not function properly. What is an intriguing possibility, though, is it's possible that there was a spontaneous hemorrhage and then you became altered because of that.

DR. JOHN CARIDI: It's always possible that you blacked out for one reason or another. If you had some kind of underlying seizure disorder or your electrolytes were screwed up, it's not inconceivable. But it's unlikely that you would just collapse. In order to collapse and hit your head this hard, you pretty much have to go completely limp and bang your head on something. If a wall is concrete, maybe. [Note: The walls and floor of the bar were indeed made of concrete.] You would have to completely lose all your motor control and flop.

The idea of an assault is not inconceivable because it did kind of look like somebody hit you really hard in the back of the head with something.

SONIA: Dr. Caridi did seriously ask me if you had been assaulted.

DAD: I don't think any of the people we talked to at the bar were hiding anything.

Your mom was very negative about the visit. She didn't want to go.

MOM: I don't know how the paramedics got you up those stairs. It was a terrible, terrible place.

DAD: It completed the picture of almost everything except for how the thing happened to begin with. There was nothing to see that indicated that an injury of your scale could have taken place. There was, far as I could tell, nothing that could have done the kind of damage that was done to you. Nothing.

MOM: It was always a huge question: *How did this happen? Why does he have this kind of injury? I mean, okay, maybe he was drunk and he fell down, but you don't have an injury like that where you rip your head apart.* One of the doctors did say it was more consistent with an assault. I guess you could conjure up something where somebody was out to get Drew Magary and whacked him over the head.

DAD: I don't see how even someone attacking you would have been possible. If you think you were alone in that dark hallway, it looks like somebody might've mistaken you for someone else and was trying to kill you. I can't figure out what could have caused such a grievous injury in such a space. The only dangerous element was a hard concrete floor.

DR. DAVID HELLER: The reigning theory at the time was that hallway was so narrow that you had hit your head on the wall on the way down while falling, then hit your head again on the floor.

SUSIE BANIKARIM: There had been this assumption that maybe there had been some condition that caused you to fall. Like a brain tumor. When you came out of surgery, the doctor clarified that hadn't been the case. You had had an injury in the front and the back of your head. Why would you have had both injuries? I think the hard part was accepting that there may not be a satisfying answer to any of that.

DR. DAVID HELLER: I would venture a pretty strong guess that this was far bigger than most of these hematomas are and that your odds of surviving were much lower than fifty-fifty.

DR. JOHN CARIDI: Every fiber of my being believes that this was not spontaneous. Something happened.

THE FOG

I was still awake, but that was about all that could be said about me at the time. So much of me was still missing, physically and otherwise. I had lost over 30 pounds while I was under. I know this because my hospital bed had its own scale built in. When I arrived in New York to host the Deadspin Awards, I weighed 220 pounds. When they turned on the bed scale, I was down to a feeble 188. I do not recommend this approach toward weight loss.

I got severely light-headed while standing and was considered a fall risk. A dickish fall risk. That meant I was not medically cleared to walk, piss, or shower unattended. If I violated those directives, I could fall on the floor and we'd have to go through the whole near-death thing all over again.

For my first attempt at standing, they strapped me to a gurney and tilted it vertically, Hannibal Lecter style. They wheeled me down the hall and I shouted that I was uncomfortable and wanted to be put down again. The nurses urged me to stay upright for as long as I could. I didn't want to hear it. I felt nauseous. Dizzy. Unmoored. I just wanted to lie down forever so that I wouldn't feel like shit. I kept yelling that I didn't like being upright. I wanted everyone to leave me the fuck alone, which is a strange desire to have when you've just been yanked back from the abyss. But I had it all the same. I was growing less erratic, but with that increased lucidity came a hefty dose of anger. My lack of gratitude was its own exhausting mystery.

SONIA: You were in a step-down unit and you kept asking people for Miller Lite. I would always talk to the doctors to be like, *He's saying all this stuff. It doesn't make any sense. Can you lessen whatever drugs he's on?* I felt like it was my job to question them. Nobody else was doing that.

JESSE: You were asking for us to bring you shitty beer, and you wanted wasabi peas.

SONIA: You were so thirsty. So we got you ice-cold seltzer from the deli. We were bringing you outside food too, because you wouldn't touch the hospital food.

HOWARD: It was really sad seeing your mom trying to get you to eat the plainest possible food. You were pushing it away. Your mom was like, *No, you gotta eat it.* Like a small child being fed by their mother.

ERICA: The first time I went to see you, I was shocked and scared because you were so skinny. Emaciated. Holocaust victim skinny. I knew that you were at least awake, but now it was like, *Well, who's inside?*

HOWARD: It was shocking to see how thin you'd gotten. You always had a big head. So you had this giant head on this scrawny, scrawny body.

ERICA: Noise was hard for you. You were super irritated, and that didn't feel like you.

MATT UFFORD: You were trying to get up to introduce me to your father. You're incoherent and pointing to me and your dad, trying to do introductions despite being the person least well equipped to do it in the room. You called me Mark, and you wanted to send me out for beer, seltzer, and peanuts.

AMANDA: Somebody brought you a huge bottle of whiskey when you were inanimate, like *what the fuck?* Sonia was like, *Get that outta here. That needs to be gone.*

SCOTT (the one who brought the whiskey): There was a point after I walked out of your room after that first visit where I did that TV movie move where the overwhelmed protagonist slides slowly down the hospital wall, head in hands, and then cries. This was back when Howard was telling me they weren't sure you'd ever fully recover full brain function and whatnot. You spent most of the night trying to steal my phone and commanding me to go to the store to buy you beer. And I was crying because of you, and your family and kids and all the other horrible things it would mean if you didn't make it all the way back.

SONIA: I did consider getting you Miller Lite. [Laughs.] I told the staff I wanted to do anything to make you happy. And they were like, *No.*

You went from the ICU to a room with four beds and curtains again. I remember the guy across from you. He was in a bad way. He was convulsing and drooling. And I was like, *Oh, man.* That's when you were asking for the beer and you thought the hospital was on rails. I was just happy you were talking, but it was not making any sense.

ERICA: You recognized who I was. You were getting kind of excited. *You're going to get me out. I have to get out of here. Help me up.* And I was like, *What are you talking about?* You tried to throw one of your legs over the bed. Your dad was on one side and had to reposition your leg back.

Sonia was like, *Drew, what the fuck are you doing? You can't go anywhere.* She was angry at you. It was the anger of somebody who is scared and wants what's best for you, but also frustrated because it's like, *Why are you doing something so stupid?*

ALEX: You always wanted seltzer and you always wanted your phone, and you wanted to get back to work. You felt like you'd been lying around and just wasting time. *What am I doing in here? Why am I still pissing around in this place? I have important things I need to be doing. I should just get up and leave and go.*

BARRY PETCHESKY: A few days before Christmas we brought sixty dollars' worth of Korean food, which was a waste ultimately. Because you opened it while we were there and had a couple of bites, but then you decided you weren't hungry anymore. You were yourself, but still understated. Forty percent less you.

MEGAN GREENWELL: Barry and I, oh my God, we got so much fucking Korean food for you. But you seemed not normal. You really wanted tea. And so we went down to the cafeteria to get you tea, but the cup was hot and full and you were lying down and you couldn't drink the tea. It was a disaster. You were mad at this tea thing, because they wanted you to be drinking things and you had to sit up to drink things. But you were so mad because only lying flat felt good. And so you were complaining, complaining, complaining. In a way that was not normal.

SONIA: I bought you a banana pudding cupcake. Brought it all the way across town to the hospital so you could enjoy it. You took two bites and didn't want the rest.

AMANDA: I remember there was all this football on TV, and you're totally out of it and you didn't care. I was like, *Oh crap, he's really not* *doing well.* I was telling you what was happening. It's fucking sad when *I'm* telling *you* about football. Then you got more interested in it. That was like, *Oh, he might be okay.*

DAD: There was some concern amongst us in general during the last week you were in the hospital, before you were released, about your temperament. You were expressing negative feelings, let's put it that way.

AMANDA: You were just saying wacky stuff. But then you got on the phone with Sonia, and the minute you got on with her, you're like, *Woof, woof* to Carter. I was crying. I was so relieved when you did that, because you were doing all the little things that make you you. That made me hysterically cry. You're like, *Where are you, Sonia? Come here, Sonia.* You kept asking where Sonia was, and you were remembering the kids' names.

SONIA: When you were lying in the rehab hospital, I gave you headphones. Do you remember this? [Note: I do not.] You asked for headphones to listen to music. And then you're like, *These are busted.* I said, *They're brand new.* You said, *I can't hear anything out of this ear.* We asked the doctors about it and they were like, *That could be a side effect. We don't really know.*

You didn't like PT. We had to get you in a wheelchair. At some point you progressed to a walker, but you had to have someone behind you and you didn't like that. You always wanted to do things yourself. You didn't want anybody in the bathroom. You didn't want anybody with you in the shower. Meanwhile, if you slipped and fell, it would be back to square one, which you didn't understand. The first picture I took of you at PT, your mouth was open. You were trying to do a puzzle. And I was like, *Oh, that's bad. We've got some work to do.* And then you would do it. I can't remember if I had to give you a pep talk or not. The doctor was adamant about you sitting up and doing stuff. He was not flexible, which is why your mom and I didn't like him. He was right, though.

DAD: We kept wondering if you were going to get tired of us.

VICTOR JEFFREYS: I remember seeing you and thinking all you wanted to do was move your body. Your body was tired of lying there. I don't know how much you move around in general, but I remember thinking, *His body hates being on its back for this amount of time.* I'm sure bodies don't like that experience.

ERICA: Sonia was very calm. Not as calm as your parents were, but she made a joke about how, when this was all over, you were gonna have to get her a really big piece of fucking jewelry because of all the stress. *He's going to pay me back big time.*

CHRISTMAS

2018

In my clearing mind, I was gonna get back home before Christmas. I would see Carter again. To this day, the kids insist that Carter is the best gift they've ever been given. Flora still says adopting him was the happiest day of her life, and she says it with the kind of conviction you *never* hear out of a teenager. It was one of the happiest days of *my* life, too. Now I missed my dog dearly. I thought we'd be reunited before the holiday.

But I was getting light-years ahead of myself, suffering delusions of the more earthly variety. There would be no Christmas back in Maryland. Santa had already given the kids all of their big gifts—a PS4 included—earlier in the month anyway. St. Nick was no fool. The kids needed a reason to feel cheery, and a free PlayStation does that trick nicely. For actual Christmas, I was stuck.

And I wasn't alone.

I had been transferred to the physical rehab ward. I was in a double and had a succession of three roommates. The first and the third roommates were fine. The second roommate was a suckling pig to Mephistopheles. He was a former NYPD detective from Staten Island who told every fucking person who showed up in the room that he was a former NYPD detective from Staten Island. I'll call him

Larry because he sounded like a Larry. Larry berated the hospital staff constantly. One night, they ushered Larry into the bathroom to have a bowel movement, and I heard him scream at the nurse, "I don't need anyone watchin' me do dis, LEAST OF ALL YOU!" I'd tell you that I would feel personally insulted if someone told me, point blank, that I wasn't qualified to watch an elderly man take a dump. But then again, who IS qualified for such duties?

I was the only patient in my ward who managed to poop in silence. Not Larry. Larry sounded like he was shitting out a live rat. It didn't matter that it was the middle of the night and the rest of us were trying to sleep. This man still made an unholy racket. At one point I heard him tell the staff, "I'm not complainin'. I'm not complainin'. BUT I WILL FILE MY FORMAL COMPLAINT TOMORRUH!" I should have filed a formal complaint about his formal complaint. He also somehow ended up wearing one of my T-shirts without realizing it was my T-shirt. Sonia got it back and wanted to burn it.

As Larry pissed and moaned, I noticed that the hearing in my right ear was struggling. I snapped my fingers by the ear to test it but couldn't tell how bad the damage was. I brought the issue up to a doctor, and he assured me that whatever hearing loss I had suffered was likely the result of my concussion, and that it would come back in due course. In the meantime, I could mute the bulk of the noise around me, Larry included, by turning on my left side, with my good ear smothered by the pillow. It was a neat little trick.

One day, Larry was finally transferred out of our room to his own single. Hopefully he didn't tear-gas any protesters along the way. Realizing Larry was gone from the room was easily the best Christmas present I received.

Meanwhile, my occupational therapist, Lucinda, came to my room and scheduled me for my twice-daily appointments in the rehab gym at the end of the ward. I lifted tiny weights, arranged cones on a shelf, did logic problems, and exercised on an arm cycle.

The arm cycle was pure evil. Two minutes on it and I was begging for stillness. I also needed lessons on how to get in and out of a shower and how to use a toilet without falling, which involved Lucinda taking me to the head and then having me sit up and down from a real toilet while keeping my pants on.

To sharpen my mind, Lucinda had me fill out hypothetical daily planners, like I was back out in the real world again. She tested my memory using flash cards and had me do basic number patterns. From there, things got trickier. I had to listen to her list off fifteen words ("house . . . monkey . . . dingleberry . . .") and then recite as many of them back to her as I could remember. I had to count down from one hundred as fast as I could. She gave me a word category, and I had to reel off as many words as I could think of that fit that category off the top of my head. Even if you haven't suffered brain damage, go ahead and list as many animals as you can think of. Once you leave the pet store and the barnyard, it suddenly gets dicier. Then, as a final gauntlet, I again had to recite as many words from the original list of fifteen as I could recall. I fiercely attempted to *win* these tests, both to impress myself and to get an early discharge. I was very proud when I did well on them. I felt like I had just won a pizza party for my grade-school class. Maybe Mitch could come.

I was coming back into myself again, albeit with a slowness I was only beginning to comprehend. I could stay upright for longer stretches, but I still succumbed to both nausea and vertigo at the end of every attempt. I dreaded OT even though I knew I needed it. Lucinda, like my doctors, told me that I had to spend as much time sitting up as humanly possible. When she caught me flat on my back in my bed, she scolded me for it.

"You're not gonna get out of here if you don't keep at it," she reminded me. "I can't say this in front of the rest of the group, but you're the only patient on this floor who's gonna get his life back. And you're not gonna get that life back if you don't work at it.

You'll just be here forever." Lucinda's job was not to give me warm fuzzies. She was motivating me to get back to the life I had so that I could make the best of it, because not everyone gets that chance.

I had no choice but to obey her, even though I hated to.

SONIA: There was one week left before Christmas vacation. I was like, *Fuck it. The kids aren't going to learn anything.* I emailed the schools to tell them that the kids weren't coming. I shut the house down, paid the bills that I could, and we went back up.

AMANDA: I just could not get into Christmas.

MOM: Your dad and I decorated the Airbnb. Howard brought over a little Charlie Brown tree. It was very sweet. Alex came back at some point and strung the lights on the tree.

SONIA: There was a fireplace with a mantel and then a little bay window on the corner where the Christmas tree was.

AMANDA: We used to like to look out that window at all the cars below and the decorations. It was intensely bright: horrible LED lighting everywhere. It made me want to barf. Every light imaginable was on, and it was really weird.

SONIA: I brought a couple of Christmas books and was just crying when I was reading to the boys. And then, a couple of days later, Rudy said, "It's too much." He had a breakdown. "I feel overwhelmed" is what he said.

AMANDA: I decorated for Christmas. We went to Paper Source, and Mom got these Christmas crafts that were in a hundred fucking pieces. There were tiny triangles that you were supposed to fit together to create a mermaid swimming through the ocean. So I spent a lot of time doing that.

Mom wanted candles. She wanted everything to look nice for Sonia, to create some normalcy. Because at that point we didn't know how long we were going to be there. I go to these stores and, like, there were little votive candles for like sixty dollars. I'm like, *Screw that.* I bought Hanukkah candles for fifty cents each. Howard brought over a tree with little lights and he was like, *Uh, sorry, I'm not really the best at decorating trees. You can never count on a Jew to string Christmas lights on a tree.*

SONIA: It was a very sad Christmas. I mean, it was happy in some ways. We were still together. We tried to decorate your room. You seemed very depressed. You seemed not happy to see us. I didn't take it personally. I knew that you still had a cocktail of drugs going through you. God knows what that does. I just figured you were miserable being there. You wanted to get out.

HOWARD: I think it was tiring for you to talk to people.

BYRD LEAVELL: I had conflicting emotions, because you were a difficult patient. Everyone was so happy you lived. You were dead. Fucking dead. But now they had this irate person that was in an early phase of recovery.

SONIA: The tough part about Christmas to New Year's is the staff thins out. You would have gone home a week or so earlier if it had been during another time. They needed a break, and I get that. But it puts you in a tough spot, and I was so pushy. I can't even tell you. I'm like, *Why isn't the PT happening today? Let's do that.*

MOM: Toward the end, oh, we were all just dying to get home. Poor little Colin, he was crying. *I want to go home, I want my room, I want my dog.*

I was so proud of you when you were in that rehab, because it was very painful and you wanted to get home and you worked hard. You really did.

ERICA: Sonia was almost in shock by how fast in some ways you were recovering. It seemed to be truly defying the odds.

Indeed, after two weeks in and out of a coma and another three weeks learning to live upright again, I got a discharge date of January 8. I was officially stable enough to leave the hospital. I was gonna go home.

SAMER KALAF: The part that I'll take away is that like everybody came together and reacted appropriately. Everybody was on top of their game. It was a situation that needed to be handled immediately to save your life.

JESSE: Everybody in your family was super together, united, *We're going to tackle this.*

ALEX: I haven't thought about this stuff in so long, because I don't want to. I want to forget. To pretend like it never happened. Fortunately you're doing so well that it's kind of *easy* to pretend. But thank God you recovered the way you did.

MOM: You said, and I remember this, "My brain is working the way I want it to now, Mom." That was enough for me.

MATT UFFORD: There's a hard division between nearly losing your life and the life that comes after. Your life could have ended at forty-two. You wouldn't have seen your kids. You wouldn't have been able to hug or kiss your wife again. Every day that you get to do that is just gravy now. You've gotten free life.

ERICA: I have to be the one to die first, because I can't deal with anybody around me dying. I can't deal with that kind of sadness again.

MOM: This is part of you now. Part of your experience. You've got the scars to show it. It's what's going to make you Drew going forward.

SONIA: Don't ever do that again.

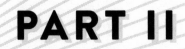

PART II

HOME

I t's not easy to transport a 195-pound man who has only half a brain, limited vestibular function, and a lingering desire to remain flat when he's afforded the luxury. Sonia looked into getting me back to Maryland in the back of an ambulance, hopefully with a speedier EMT at the wheel. Sticker price was $8,000. Insurance covered the bulk of my brain surgery ($70,000) but scoffed at shelling out a penny more to get my ass home. She thought about driving me back in our car but didn't trust herself for the job. I wasn't allowed to fly. Amtrak was also out, because those trains rattle way more than you think (pissing in an Amtrak bathroom is like shooting clay pigeons, only less of a rush) and because walking through Penn Station on a Tuesday certainly won't DECREASE brain damage.

Enter Byrd Leavell. Byrd lived in New York. Byrd had a car. Byrd was willing to drive us to Maryland that morning, then drive himself back home, all in one day. He did not ask for an extra cut of sales from this book for the offer.

Also, we were gonna stop for Popeyes. I needed Popeyes like it was a bonus shot of fentanyl.

The morning of my discharge, an attendant named Dwight walked into my hospital room and looked over my chart. To insurers, my medical history now reads like a rap sheet. Doctors had signed my discharge papers the night before. My getaway was a done deal, as far as I was concerned.

"I'm still getting out today, right?" I asked Dwight.

"Actually, nah, there's been a slight delay."

"There has?"

"I'm just messin' around. Yeah, you're out today."

I wanted to be like *Don't toy with me, Dwight,* but I was too relieved that he was kidding to say an unkind word. In fact, I was still under the impression that I had been a good patient all these weeks. After all, I had made a point of learning every nurse's name and thanking them every time they gave me a shot of heparin at four in the morning. I wasn't like Larry. I was a nice guy.

But I wasn't. I had been a seething mess the whole time I was in the hospital. All I wanted was silence and privacy. Hospitals are not engineered for either of these things, nor are they supposed to be. I seethed at loud doctors making speakerphone calls from just outside my room. I openly snapped at the staff members who had to keep vigil over me at night while I slept, and while I pissed, and even while I showered. These doctors and staffers saved my life. They were never anything but kind and protective toward me, and yet I resented them. I pretended to nap sometimes when my parents visited, so that they would go away and leave me be. I don't know why I did that. All they wanted was to see their son alive. Whatever darkness had enveloped me the night of my hemorrhage was still there, poisoning my soul.

Then Dwight confirmed my discharge and I became convinced that I could leave all of that darkness behind. Mom, Dad, and Sonia came up to my room as Dwight loaded me into a wheelchair and I got a final look at both my room and the rehab ward of Mount Sinai. My bed would not stay unoccupied for long.

Dwight took us down to the lobby, and the first thing I noticed was it was fucking cold. I had been freezing in my room, likely due to the fact that I had shed my usual layer of protective winter blubber while comatose. The vestibule to the lobby was even colder. The automatic hospital doors opened every five seconds to let in both new patients and a fresh blast of January. New York is one of those cities where the cold is ruder. It does not make you tougher or stronger to brave the New York cold. It makes you BITCHIER. *Who's the asshole who let all this cold into town?* That kind of cold.

A vestibule acts as a terrestrial spaceship hatch: a holding area to let people from the street in without exposing people in the main lobby to the nasty elements outside. It's roughly as comfortable as a bus stop. But I was out of my room, so I could deal. I was sitting on a bench with my dad, mere feet away from finally being back out in the relatively fresh air (I was still in New York, mind you; the hospital didn't exit out to an empty pasture). I was ready to go.

Byrd was stuck in traffic. The doors opened and shut. Opened and shut. Opened and shut. I thought about going back into the main lobby for a slight boost in warmth, but it wasn't worth having my view of the outside world obscured further. Also, I was in that zone where you're waiting for a car—be it in the city, or at the airport, or outside of school, or at a hotel—and you think the next car passing is your ride, only it turns out to be some asshole in a Camry. Every car you see raises your hopes and then flattens them in a single pass. All the non-Byrd cars could go to hell, as far as I was concerned.

Finally Byrd arrived. Dwight wheeled me over to the passenger side, helped me up, and then loaded me into the car like the bulk cargo that I was. I rolled down the window and gave Mom and Dad a final goodbye. We were going our separate ways, but it's not exactly like it was a bittersweet parting. It had been a long, long month for my parents. They wanted to go back home as badly as I did.

"We love you, Drew," Mom said. "Safe travels. Do what Sonia says."

Sonia insisted that I sit up for the entire ride. Both of us were unsure if I could withstand the rigors of the Jersey Turnpike, but Sonia had long since adopted Lucinda's stance that I needed to be up more if I wanted to *stay* up. Once I got into Byrd's car, I instantly violated that order by reclining my seat to an obnoxious 135-degree angle. I figured that was upright enough. She allowed it.

We left Manhattan through the dreaded Lincoln Tunnel, the same way Sonia and I had moved out of the city back on New Year's Eve of 2003. She had always wanted to move back to Maryland, since she was from there. I had always resisted, since I didn't know anyone in that area. But Sonia's the shrewd negotiator, talented at extracting concessions from anyone, including our own stubborn offspring. By contrast, I am the world's shittiest negotiator. I don't even have the balls to return big-ticket items at a department store because I fear a floor manager's rejection. It wasn't me who returned that solar watch back to the Macy's counter. Sonia did. She could have gotten her money back without a receipt, or a tag, or an ID, or even without the fucking watch itself. She could return our children if we needed to. Always good to have that chit handy.

We packed up a U-Haul that New Year's with help from Sonia's cousin, who would himself suffer a catastrophic brain injury after falling off a cliff (!!!) in Greece while on assignment for CNN in 2008. Our combined blood lineage has not been good to heads. Sonia cried when we left New York all those years ago, which always amused me because *I* was the one who didn't want to leave.

But there was no crying this time around. We were ready to get the fuck out.

"Do you mind if I take a business call?" Byrd asked while driving. I did not. For once I would get to listen to someone besides a doctor take a call on speakerphone. I would get to hear the normal comings and goings of the world as I had remembered them.

Byrd mentioned to his associate that he was driving us, and I felt that weird sense of misplaced pride people get when someone else name-drops them on the phone. I wanted to voice-bomb the call. I wanted to be like, *YEAH, SONIA AND I ARE HERE TOO! I BELIEVE MY BRAIN NEEDS NO INTRODUCTION!*

I did not do that. Instead, I looked out the window and thought about fried chicken.

The view of the Jersey Turnpike, underwhelming under any other circumstance, was majestic on this day. I got a front-row view of Newark airport, the oil refineries, the IKEA in Elizabeth, the signs that tell you that the next rest stop is 782 miles ahead, and the end of the turnpike split, where cars and trucks merge back together and South Jersey becomes the middle of nowhere. It was beautiful.

We crossed over the Delaware Memorial Bridge and into a tiny state that exists mainly to shake down cars passing through for exorbitant tolls to lard its coffers. But Delaware did have a lovely rest area, with both a Popeyes *and* a self-serve gas station. Pre-COVID, Jersey had only full serve, because it wanted you to suffer.

The weather was relatively mild for January. The rest area had tables and benches outside for anyone who wanted to dine alfresco and watch Mayflower trucks barreling past at ninety miles per hour in either direction. Yet another majestic sight. But I remained colder than stone, so we went inside. I had been dreaming about this chicken for days, if not weeks. This was gonna be my first meal back out in civilization, and I would get to enjoy it inside a rest-area pavilion with a thousand of the Northeast Corridor's finest meth-addled drivers. Byrd and I sat at a table while Sonia volunteered to grab the food.

"You had to take a shit," Byrd remembers of the stop. "I was like, *Wow, we are* really *friends now,* because I had to help you walk there.

"There was this other moment I felt was significant. You looked at me and you said, 'Byrd, I don't remember anything. I woke up and I don't remember a single goddamn thing.' That was a moment of clarity between us."

It was true. During my hospital stay, I lived in a netherworld between full consciousness and drug-addled mirages, so it's hard to pinpoint when I regained full control of my mind. The whole timeline is a loose pile of glass shards on a floor. Even the moment I "woke up," with the nurse telling me I had been in a coma, was just one instance of my coming in and out of lucidity along the sedation continuum. The where and the when and the what of that encounter are all as ephemeral as a fresh dream. Worst of all, I had no idea that I was hallucinating *while* I was hallucinating. So my memory of recovering at Mount Sinai is a clutter of real events along with delusions so real and so vivid that my mind has no ability to distinguish between the two. I remembered a detailed conversation with Megan Greenwell and David Heller in my room about my injury that Megan insists, quite credibly, never happened. I would go on to debate the existence of this conversation with her for *months*.

Sonia brought the food back to our table. She had gotten tenders instead of bone-in chicken. I was crushed. I really wanted the *chicken* chicken. But I held my tongue. Sonia had just endured hell on earth, popping Xanax and crying herself to sleep every night as she labored to get me out of that hospital. Besides, I was hungry, and any chicken tender is a good chicken tender. It was my job to shut the fuck up, although I would shirk those duties as I regained my strength.

Get your life back. That was the idea. That was the miracle I was gunning for. Not quite getting the fast food order I was craving fit in perfectly with my old lifestyle. This is not a world waiting to please you. Just as I had prayed that Colin would grow old enough to irritate me when he was clinging to life as a preemie in the

NICU (after his birth, he was hospitalized for a full month), I now hoped that I could take my own life for granted once again. I was prepared for the opportunity. Too much so.

Another two hours in the car and we were finally at the Chez Magary doorstep, just outside of DC. Flora, Rudy, and Colin came running out the door to give me hugs and kisses. Before I arrived, they had made a giant WELCOME HOME DAD! sign, complete with colored-in hearts and smiley faces and the name "Dad" written inside the contours of every enclosed letter. They forgot to hang it up on the door before I came, but that didn't matter. I wept at the sight of it. I have the sign framed behind my computer right now, as I'm typing this. I should look at it more often. Closely. Not just let it linger in my periphery. I should remind myself, with much greater frequency, not only how happy I was to be home but how happy *they* were for me to return.

Carter included. Back at the hospital, Colin had said to me, "Carter's gonna wag his tail so hard when he sees you, he's gonna fly." When Carter is pumped, he wags his tail in a vigorous circular motion, not unlike a helicopter's rotor blades. When I walked back inside the house for the first time in over a month, Carter wasn't airborne, but goddamn if he wasn't putting his best effort into it. Everyone else in my family knew what had happened to me and knew that I was going to live. But Carter had been in the dark the entire time. All he knew was that I walked out the door one December morning, possibly for a pack of cigarettes, and then never came back. This is the kind of doggy ignorance that owners like me typically envy. I'm always like, *Hey, I'd like to be a dog so I can lick my own ass and snack on jerky treats all day.* But in this case, Carter had no idea where I'd been, or what had happened, or if I'd ever come back. He was in a waking coma of his own.

So when he laid eyes on me, he was *elated*. Shaking with happiness. And Carter isn't the most affectionate of dogs. In fact, Carter was so rough around the edges after we brought him home in 2016 that he bit Sonia and me, drawing blood. His growls were not playful growls. He'd get angry without warning and lash out at us. We worried he might bite the kids. Or other kids. Or anyone else who had unwittingly drawn his ire. All we wanted to do was love this dog, but the stress of *living* with him got to the point where we thought long and hard about taking him back to the shelter.

But we never did. We never could. The kids loved him too much, and so did I. We got Carter a trainer and, with time and effort, he mellowed out. But he remains aloof in certain ways. He only gives kisses to Colin, and Colin has to put his eye within a millimeter of Carter's mouth to get a lick. The rest of us have to settle for sniffs. He demands tummy rubs but not once has he ever given ME one, which seems lopsided. He'll only jump on your lap if you bribe him with cheese. And if you pet him when he's not in the mood, he's like, *The fuck you doing?*

But when I sat down in my recliner the day I got home, Carter jumped onto me and nestled into my lap like he had been waiting to do so for a month. And maybe he had. No cheese bribe required. I petted him and stifled a tear. He was, as ever, soft as a lamb. Insane dog people *love* to interpret their dog's thoughts in their favor. It's one of the perks of owning a dog. In reality a dog is just thinking, *That's the asshole who eats a steak right in front of me and won't gimme any. I'll piss on his shoes.* But now I got to indulge myself and put words in Carter's mouth. *DREW! DREW IS BACK! I LOVE HIM I LOVE HIM I LOVE HIM I LOVE HIM I LOVE HIM.*

I was tired. I had just left a hospital after a traumatic brain injury and traveled through four states with no guarantee that I would survive the trip without throwing up, fainting, or accidentally bashing my head getting out of Byrd's car. The ride back was all so familiar and yet still a lot to absorb. As such, my recliner wasn't reclining enough. I needed to lie down.

As in the hospital, lying down was a physically and psychologically unwise thing to do. Oh, but it didn't *feel* unwise. It felt like the smartest idea in history to my ailing soul. Yes, I *could* stay up and feel seasick and listen to everyone in the house be way too loud. Was it me or had everyone gotten *louder* in my absence? Or I could decamp upstairs to a comfy, comfy bed. It would be like my hospital bed, only good! Who was I to resist its siren call? It was a quality bed. It had fluffy pillows and everything. And my discharge instructions mandated that I rest, did they not?

Sonia gave me the go-ahead. Carter jumped off my lap and she helped me upstairs so I could lie down in my own bed for the first time since 2018. Whatever the coma did to me, it did not make me afraid of sleeping. I did not close my eyes in abject terror that they would never again open. My coma had been kind. Perhaps too kind, given the external havoc it had wreaked. I had no hesitation about returning to the black.

So I slept, this time for one hour and one hour only. After that, I was up again and ready to live.

Somewhat.

THE ROAD TO NORMAL

I wasn't allowed to drive, exercise, travel long distances, climb the stairs unaccompanied, walk in socks on a hardwood floor, work, or even take ibuprofen for pain. My job was to stay home and give my brain time to rest (though not exclusively with sleep). To heal at its own speed. I was effectively quarantined, which gave me a nice dry run for the worldwide quarantine that would come just over a year later. As you are now intimately aware, quarantine BLOWS. Instead of being stuck in a hospital, I was stuck at our place, which was a decided upgrade from Mount Sinai but still meant I was living apart from the outside world. Our house had become my halfway house.

Sonia had extra railings installed along the staircase and even in the shower. She toyed with the idea of a stair lift, but stair lifts cost a fortune and I refused to be stair-lift years old. She also bought a shower stool at the behest of the hospital staff, and I hated it with an intense fury. But I was still a fall risk, and shower floors are hard. Thus, Sonia insisted I sit down when delousing myself. I never used it, except whenever she caught me standing in there. Then I would sit down, wait for her to leave the bathroom, and stand right back up again.

In the shower, I discovered the surreal dermatological effects that result from prolonged unconsciousness. If you suffer from dry skin during the winter, like I do, a coma does not help matters. My heels looked like fucking dinosaur eggs. On the plus side, I couldn't bite my nails while I was under, so when I woke up they looked better than they had in *years*. Sonia had a pumice stone in the shower that I used to grind my leathery feet back down into something more closely resembling human appendages. It would take more than one session—many more—with that stone to complete the sanding and buffing process.

I also had a walker. Two walkers, actually: one for upstairs and one for the main floor. The downstairs one could venture outside, although navigating weather-beaten roads with a walker is a Tik-Tok waiting to happen. The upstairs one was for venturing to the toilet whenever I wanted to piss in the middle of the night. I have a weak bladder and always get up to piss at night. I also toss. I turn. I scratch my face *constantly*. I rub the whites of my eyes. It's like sleeping with a chimp.

Sonia treasures sleep like it's her fourth child, so I have to get up gingerly during my nighttime pissing excursions to keep from waking her. I don't even turn the light on when I go. I rely exclusively on my urinary sonar. But after getting out of the hospital, I had to introduce a walker to the ritual. *You* try grabbing for a walker in the dark at 3:00 A.M. and scooting it along the floor without making a sound. You'd have to be a fucking magician to pull this off. Sonia outfitted the front legs of the walker with cut tennis balls—Florida style—to reduce the noise and to prevent scratches on the floors. Didn't matter. The circus still came to town whenever I got up to piss. If I knew Sonia was deep asleep, I ditched the walker and made the trip without it. But she always knew. Nothing got by her, nor does it still.

"You went to the bathroom last night without the walker," she told me one morning.

I rolled my eyes like I was Flora. "I know, I know."

"I am *not* going through all that again."

"Copy that."

I used the walker at all times after that, keeping it by my side like a second dog. The trick to using a walker—and you'll need this tip when you turn seventy-five—is that you can't lean on it. That sounds counterintuitive, but if you put all your body weight on the walker, not only will you eat the curb if it gets away from you, but you'll grow a hump on your back the size of an angel food cake. I did not grow that hump, but I got my old-man shuffle down to perfection. In fact, during my initial stages of recovery, I acquired a few other tics usually reserved for elderly shuffleboard enthusiasts. I played a lot of sudoku. I sat down to put on my undies. I had a pillbox! The one Sonia bought me was circular, which made it much younger and cooler than the miniaturized ice cube tray your grandpa uses to take his Lipitor every day. In the span of less than two months, I had aged thirty years.

Twice a week I got a house call from an occupational therapist named Sharene, who tested my mental dexterity, my movement, and my balance. I had to walk in a straight line, heel to toe, to my front door and back. A field sobriety test, in essence. I did not succeed on my first effort, nor on my second. Sharene walked alongside me to keep me upright if I stumbled, and I stumbled more than a few times.

"Did the hospital give you a cane?" she asked me.

"No. Do I get one?"

"You may want to use one instead of a walker."

"Hell yeah, I would." I envisioned strutting around town with a lacquered mahogany cane and a pocket watch to go with it, taking my rightful place as an underground mafia kingpin.

"Let me bring you a cane next session and see how it works for you."

She brought a cane for me to sample, but it was one of those orthopedic canes with a square base, like it had a tiny walker attached to the end of it. Not a pimp cane. I would still look like an old fart. More important, the cane wasn't useful. I might as well have been walking around with a couple of cinched umbrellas. It was the walker or nothing.

Sharene's visits represented peak excitement that January. A few friends did check in on me that month, including Susie Banikarim, Gabe Fernandez, Chris Thompson, and my boss at Deadspin before Megan Greenwell, Tim Marchman. This is what happens when you grow old. You don't throw keggers. You have visits: people popping in for a quick talk and maybe a light snack before they go back about their day. I made little avocado toasts for everyone, like a fancy boy, and then ate half of them myself.

I couldn't entertain my old friends for very long. After just ten minutes, I was exhausted. Again, the visitors seemed too loud. Had everyone always been so loud? Also, I was still freezing. All the time. I was in bed by 8:00 P.M. every night, with the comforter stapled to my chin. It was pathetic. One night I ate ice cream and had to stop because the ice cream itself was making my whole body so fucking cold. If my body temp didn't improve, I was gonna have to spend every night sleeping inside a freshly opened bear carcass.

The rest of that month involved me sitting in my chair, bored out of my mind. I texted Megan Greenwell, begging her to let me go back to work. Brain surgery or not, writing has always helped me piece my mind together. It's how I complete my thoughts. I had a computer on a standing desk—okay, the desk is a table with a chair on top of it—in the office, and I was dying to use it. I don't like things getting in the way of me writing, and the hemorrhage was proving to be a stubborn barrier. In fact, that's one of the few things I remember distinctly from my postcoma fog at the hospital. I remember feeling inconvenienced, as my brother Alex noticed. I was like, *Well, this is a pain in the ass. I got bowl games to write about!* Now my computer was mere feet away but Sonia, in a twist from the average CBS sitcom wife, ordered me to sit in my beloved recliner and stay lazy.

I begged her to let me write for an hour here and there, and she relented. I dragged myself over to my desk and got down notes, random paragraphs, and anything else I could before fatigue set in and I had to decamp to the bed. On a table behind my desk was a folder containing all of my medical files from the accident, which Sonia kept meticulously organized for reference. On the inside of the folder she taped the business card of every specialist who had treated me, with their phone numbers and emails circled in ink so we could contact them directly as needed.

She also kept a CaringBridge journal while I was in the hospital, which she told me was more for her sake than mine. I couldn't bring myself to read her entries, to see in her own words what she had gone through. Also, Amanda had taken a photo of me while I was in a coma and sent it to my email address in case I wanted to gawk at it. I couldn't look at that yet, either. I wasn't ready. I had done a 180 from my hospital sloth and was now interested only in moving forward and salvaging all that I had lost.

That included writing. I was skirting doctors' orders by working, and yet, at the same time, I was doing the right thing by staying upright for as long as was tolerable. Soon I was writing more, and for longer. This was me getting closer to normal. Soon I'd be working full time again and bungee jumping and climbing K2 and doing all kinds of wild shit. I also violated discharge orders by cooking earlier than I was supposed to, despite the fact that Sonia's college friends had bought us a very generous Seamless gift card to help with meals, which remains the single most useful get-well present that I have ever received. Still, no one could stop me from making myself an omelet, and Sonia was more than happy to let me indulge. I even smoked some ribs, although I was disappointed by how they'd turned out. Another time I was making dinner and grabbed a box of pasta from the cabinet that I didn't recognize.

"Where's this from?" I asked Sonia.

"From the Pioneer supermarket," she said matter-of-factly. That was the grocery store right next to their Airbnb in New York. Sonia bought that pasta to make dinner at the rental apartment while I was under. She saved it and brought it all the way back home, along with a pair of souvenir mugs from the Guggenheim Museum. Wasting that pasta would have been a crime. It deserved to live out its natural life cycle, just as all things deserve to.

No recovery has ever happened on a straight line. And yet my expectations remained unreasonable. I wanted my life back precisely as it had been. The sooner I got back to normal, the sooner I could forget that this had ever happened. All my life, I had been taught—with great evidence and great wisdom—that things happen for a reason and that you make good from bad. But I saw no good in almost dying. No one could even tell me why I had collapsed to begin with. All I saw was a miserable fluke. I wished it had never happened at all. There was nothing to learn. There was nothing about me that could be improved by enduring all this, particularly when I hadn't even been awake for the worst of it. Thus, my goal was to get back into my comfortable routines and erase the hemorrhage entirely from my personal history. According to the Centers for Disease Control and Prevention, over 1.5 million Americans suffer a traumatic brain injury (TBI) every year. I am, now and forever, one of those 1.5 million. But in January 2019, I wanted to throw my membership card for that club in a fucking fire. I didn't want to think about what happened, and I didn't want my life divided in separate epochs of Before Coma and After Coma. I wanted everything smoothed out.

Because in a perfect world, this would all be over. Everything that had passed would be left in the past. Yes, I could enjoy telling people I had almost died (you should see the look on their faces when I play that card), but I could also enjoy telling them that I had recovered fully like a big, strong man. A hemorrhage was NOTHING, baby. And by February, I was beginning to feel that way. I was no longer a fall risk. I lost the walker. I lost the dreaded shower stool. I wasn't even on meds anymore. Sonia cut my hair to even it out, and now you couldn't see my scars from the operation at all. I could brandish my trauma solely at my own discretion. If you saw me, you wouldn't have known that anything had happened to me.

But *I* knew. I could still trace a line along the scars running up the front and the back of my head. If I traced them simultaneously, my fingers almost met at the top of my scalp. When I was still at Mount Sinai, the dissolvable stitches were still there. One night, while in my hospital bed, I pulled one of them out and placed it on the bed beside my pillow. It was a coarse, wiry thing, like a whisker plucked from a small dog. For weeks, this mighty little stitch had performed the vital task of helping keep my scalp together. Once plucked, it was nothing more than biodegradable garbage. When I woke up the next morning and checked next to my hospital pillow, that stitch had vanished.

Now the wound itself almost had. Of course, that didn't stop me from picking at the scabs. Sonia reminded me over and over to leave the scabs alone, but one of them crusted over with such dependability that I couldn't help but toy with it. I am now forty-four years old and still enjoy picking scabs. When I get one off cleanly, it's satisfying in ways that should never be.

I graduated from house calls to outpatient therapy, a bittersweet achievement given that poor Sonia had to drive me to the rehab hospital for every session. She had to drive me everywhere, in fact: to the supermarket, to the drugstore, to appointments with doctors in fields I had no idea existed until I got hurt (neuro-ophthalmology!). So many appointments. Every time we visited a new specialist, the outpatient forms asked what meds I had taken after surgery and the dosage, something I had never needed to remember before. I couldn't even remember the names of some of these drugs. *How much esomeprazole was I on? Is it twenty-five milligrams? Is that right?* (It was not.) By day, Sonia worked as a preschool teacher, which was its own form of crisis management. Serving as my chauffeur only added to all of her toil. At least they gave us a temporary handicapped parking sticker.

I walked—with no assistance—into the rehab hospital for the first time and was surrounded by young and enthusiastic PTs hustling back and forth in polo shirts and stretch khakis you could run a 10K wearing. My new sensei was a short woman named Ann whose job was to up my degree of rehab difficulty. Resistance bands would be involved. If you're a casual workout person like me, the sight of resistance bands sends you fleeing in horror. Suddenly I wasn't so gung ho about being Mister Can-Do.

"Okay," Ann told me, "you're gonna tie the resistance band around your legs and walk side to side, without crossing your legs."

I did the gagged-and-bound crab walk. Every step I took, the band ripped out my precious leg hair at the root. But that was merely the opening stage of a weeks-long gauntlet that Ann put me through.

Visit number two: "I want you to take this heavy ball and bounce it against this trampoline ten times."

That was actually fun. I never dropped the ball once. *I could play for an NFL team*, I thought.

Visit three: "Now I want you to walk to the end of the ward and back while throwing this lighter ball up in the air and catching it."

That was even MORE fun. It was like field day!

Visit four: "Now I want you to stand on this balance trainer and squat down ten times."

That SUCKED. I had guardrails to keep my balance. Didn't make it any more enjoyable. Every time I had to resort to grabbing them, I felt like a failure. I wanted to go back to playing touch football with myself.

Visit five: "Now I want you to walk on this treadmill for ten minutes."

That was closer to my usual fitness routine, where I went to the gym, hopped on an elliptical trainer, and dicked around on my phone for forty-five minutes. Felt good to be back to the yuppie rituals of Before Hemorrhage Drew.

Visit six: "Now I wanna bring you over here," Ann said, escorting me to a large board with plastic buttons scattered around it. Standing before it, I felt like the captain of a spaceship built in 1982. I wanted to play with this control board badly. And guess what? I *did*.

This was a reaction-time exercise. Every time a button lit up, I had to punch it as quickly as I could. To up the stakes in the second round, I had to stare at the center of the board and recite words that appeared in a little box while, at the same time, punching the lit buttons as they appeared in my periphery. I punched the SHIT out of those buttons. I love mashing buttons as much as a baby does. When our three children were babies, I enjoyed dicking around with their toys more than they did. If they made an Exersaucer for adults, I would have bought one.

Turned out Ann had an Exersaucer of her own for me to use. But this one did NOT have bitchin' rattles or spinny things adorning it. This was a simulator designed to test my vestibular function:

my sense of balance and movement. I had done well on a lot of the exercises so far and been, characteristically, far too proud of it. The Machine was designed to crush that pride.

Ann strapped a harness on me and I stood, in my stocking feet, on a metal plate.

"For phase one, you can keep your eyes open."

"Okay." I was to look straight ahead at all times. I was allowed to grab things only if I lost my balance. Otherwise, I had to keep my hands at my sides, or else I'd be cheating.

She commenced phase one of the test, entering a bunch of information on a nearby touch screen. The metal plate under my feet quivered, then gently rolled back and forth. If you've ever been seasick, you know that the subtle movement of a boat is often worse than the big, violent shakes. I turned green. But I stayed on my feet and kept my eyes dead ahead on the Machine's brand logo as the plate grew rowdier. I survived phase one. Not a speck of vomit came out of me. Barry Petchesky would have been proud.

"For phase two, you have to close your eyes."

"Oh, God." Anytime I stood and closed my eyes after my injury, I felt drunk. And not in a fun way.

"Ready?"

"No, but go ahead."

Call this the blue-book portion of the exam. The ground beneath my feet shifted. Then quaked. Then tilted. Then spun. I was done for. I fell within seconds, with the harness the only thing keeping me from eating the ground all over again.

"I failed, huh?" I asked Ann.

Indeed, I had. My vestibular function was in the toilet. This was the aftereffect of suffering a near-lethal concussion, but there was more to it than that. I had also damaged my vision in the fall. I hadn't realized this until a neuro-ophthalmologist gave me an exam and my eyes couldn't align two glowing red lasers while looking through his spectroscope. This was but one of the many things that had gone awry inside of me and were in danger of staying that way had I left them undiagnosed and untreated.

Ann gave me reams of physical homework to do, including crab walks to my front door and back. I got a free set of resistance bands for the privilege. That's the American healthcare system for you: The only shit that's free is shit you'd NEVER want. I also had to stand on one leg in full-minute increments, first while holding on to a barstool and then free standing, if I could manage it. I had a timer on my phone set to count down the sixty seconds. Sonia thought the alarm was too loud. I told her she was being rude about it. When I did these balance and movement exercises, I took full stock of my surrounding environs to account for hard floors, sharp corners, and any other potential cranial hazards should I fall. Suddenly my house was a booby trap emporium.

I also had to draw a large dot on a sheet of paper and post it on my wall, then stand ten feet away and move my head up and down and then side to side, keeping my focus on the dot as I went. At first the dot shook and lurched. Ann told me this was normal. If I was a good boy and kept up with the exercises, the dot would gradually remain centered in my field of vision. She told me that the brain is its own electrician. "Eventually it rewires itself so that it can work around the areas that have been damaged."

"Can I drive a car again?"

"I'm afraid you're still gonna have to pass the vestibular function test."

I wasn't ready to face the Machine again just yet. But in the meantime, I was able to snatch back pieces of my old existence in a sort of reverse bucket list: I walked upright; did light home workouts; had sex again; climbed a (very small) mountain with my kids; and walked them to the bus stop and back myself.

One perfect day, I took Rudy to a soccer field to kick the ball around with him. Rudy is into soccer the way your average grandma is into cribbage. It is the center of his world. Before I got hurt, we played soccer in the yard, or in the basement if it rained. For basement soccer, we used two officially licensed NHL knee hockey goals and a tiny foam ball. Despite my age, and despite my being triple Rudy's mass, we were evenly matched on this dwarf pitch. We knew all the best angles for kicking the ball off the wall and into the net. Anytime Rudy lost to me, which wasn't often, he got *pissed,* stewing over his defeat like it had just been broadcast on national television.

Now, for the first time since I had been hospitalized, we went to a park with regulation-sized goals to stage penalty kick shoot-outs.

"Don't kick it at my head," I told Rudy.

"Okay."

That was one of those moments when my recovery adhered to cinematic expectations: a father and son enjoying a simple kick-around on a vast field. An everyday dad moment that I had nearly lost forever and now held in appropriate, purply reverence. This was what I wanted. This was the stirring comeback I had envisioned for myself. I could play with my kids again. I couldn't spin around too fast, lest I get dizzy. But I could still play.

And then we went back home and the movie cut off. I still had work to do. I had to conquer the Machine. I kept doing my exercises. I went back to rehab. Ann strapped me in. I handled phase one of the test with surprising finesse. But now came the real bitch. I shut my eyes.

"You ready?" she asked.

"Bring it."

She sicced the Machine on me. It toyed with me at first: quivers and jostles so faint, I wasn't even sure I'd moved. It's like sitting in an airplane on the tarmac and looking out the window to see if that pull you felt was the plane taxiing to the runway. Then the

Machine's footplate started doing a full Axl Rose sway. I kept my knees bent and anticipated where the footplate would tilt so that I could move in rhythm with it instead of just reacting to it. I still felt drunk, but I hung in there. After what seemed like an hour (it was ninety seconds), I lost my balance and muttered, "Shit," out loud.

"I failed, huh?"

"You did *very* well," Ann said. I didn't believe her. Physical therapists are always overly nice about your progress. They do this to keep your chin up, and also because they have to deal with a lot of stubborn jackasses who don't think PT is useful. I was a good patient now, so I didn't need to be patronized.

But Ann wasn't leading me on at all. She showed me the results. My vestibular abilities had skyrocketed. My score came in *right* below the passing threshold line on the chart.

"So I did better but I still failed? Aw, man."

"Oh, I think you're all right," she said warmly.

"I passed?"

"Technically no, but I think you're fine to get back to your usual routines now."

"Can I go to the gym?"

"Start off slow, but sure."

Nice! I still remembered the combination to my padlock to boot.

"Can I drive?"

"Yes."

"Holy shit!"

Sonia waited patiently through the bulk of these appointments, sitting in the lobby on her phone while I bounced balls and fought bravely against orthopedic sex swings. No more. She was finally liberated from driving duties. I had graduated. *We* had graduated. To celebrate, we went out for dim sum. I ate my dumplings so fast I couldn't taste them.

I was not allowed to drive home after graduation. It would not have been wise to involve the Beltway in my first attempt at operating a motor vehicle since dying. But once we got back to the house, Sonia let me drive around our neighborhood block. I was slightly nervous getting back behind the wheel. I knew I could drive; I just didn't know if doing so would trigger some brand-new vestibular dysfunction I hadn't foreseen, causing me to run over a baby.

I did not run over a baby. I gunned the engine, put my Kia in drive, and did a lap. Then I did another one just to be cocky. Driving was the same as it had always been. I could work out again too, which was good because I had been double-fisting brownies on my way to regaining twenty pounds.

And I could write full time again. A checkered flag somewhere waved in my honor. If a crowd had seen my rally, they would have roared in approval.

I just wouldn't have been able to hear them.

DEAF

My right ear wasn't getting any better. I kept snapping my fingers by the ear but couldn't tell if I was hearing anything with it or if my left ear was doing all the legwork. I visited my general practitioner—man, was it refreshing to visit an everyday doctor and *not* a doctor specializing in orthocerebrogastrohypmentiology— and he waved off the loss. "It'll come back," he reassured me. "These things just take time." It had already been months. In terms of recovery from a TBI, two months is jack shit. But YOU try living with a bum ear for that long. Ever have one ear get plugged up when you're swimming? It's fucking annoying, right? You tilt your head and jump up and down to get the water out, and the longer your ear stays plugged, the more frustrated you get. Okay, now imagine that, but forever.

I wasn't convinced by my GP. I was now old enough to know that doctors didn't know everything. When I was a kid, I assumed my pediatrician could also perform major surgery, or perhaps even stitch up a nasty head wound, in a pinch. I knew better now, brain damage or not. So I went to Dr. Kent, an ear, nose, and throat specialist (or otolaryngologist, now that we're back swimming in the medical profession's alphabet soup), and asked him about my prognosis. I was prepared for baddish news, but not for it to be delivered so swiftly and decisively.

"Oh, your hearing won't be coming back," Dr. Kent said. "You see, when you fractured your skull, the fracture tore through your inner ear."

"Can it heal?"

"Not with damage this extensive, no." He brought up an MRI of my head to show me the proof. A diagnosis of single-sided deafness (SSD) was already in my extensive medical file from Mount Sinai. But doctors there either ignored that I had pulled a Van Gogh, forgot to tell me, or were simply so determined to get me upright and back home that it wasn't high on their priority list. It wasn't high on mine while I was in there, either.

Now I could see, with improving vision, what they had ignored. It was right there on the MRI. Your brain is protected by your skull. It's a good, solid shelter for your internal hard drive. But your skull has more than a few apertures. Eighty-five of them, to be precise. These are necessary trapdoors that are the product of human evolution. They do more good than harm. But when they are compromised . . . well, that means *uh-oh* for you.

You know some of the obvious trapdoors. You have open eyeholes in your skull called orbital fissures, plus two optic canals that allow the optic nerves to carry information collected by your eyeballs through the ethmoid bones—Ethmoid Bones sounds like the name of a character from a Victorian horror story—behind them and into your brain to be interpreted as sight. Your nasal cavity is split right down the center by a mixture of bone and cartilage called the nasal septum, which gives each nostril its own doorway to your sinuses. And of course, your skull has no floor. After all, your neck and the rest of your body are already there to protect the underbelly of your head. If you had no body, then your skull would need a bottom. Let's all hope that happens when we live on as disembodied, cryogenically frozen heads later in this century.

Seeing as how these openings are, you know, *openings,* they can be breached. This is true of your nasal cavity and the underside of your jaw. These are the orifices that get penetrated with regularity in any quality action movie. But let's delve now into the more artisanal trapdoors of the human skull. Specifically, I'd like to acquaint you with the internal auditory meatus. "Meatus" is the term for any opening in the body and usually refers to the hole where urine flows out of you. Another, less comical meatus is the highway linking your outer ear—go ahead and give it a tug to let it know you're still there—to the astonishing sound factory that is your inner ear. Your outer ear is nothing more than an organic satellite dish. It captures sound from the outside, funnels it through the ol' ear meatus, and delivers it to your inner ear, where that sound is harvested, processed, packaged, and delivered to your brain as human speech, pieces of music, and loud farts.

The internal auditory meatus is located due south of the temporal bone. Men break the temporal bone three times more often than women, because breaking shit is my gender's lifelong passion. Given how hard it is to break the temporal bone, you'd be correct in assuming that, once displaced, it can break a few things of its own. In my case, the fracture tore through the meatus, cutting my inner ear off from the outside world. The inner ear and its nerve bundles assist in controlling human balance, which explained my dizziness. It also explained why I no longer had any echolocation: the ability to tell where sounds are coming from. You need both ears working to have this. Without echolocation, accidentally walking in front of an oncoming car behind you becomes a more likely occurrence.

Dr. Kent showed me all of the damage I had suffered: hairline cracks in my skull, a breached auditory canal, visible scarring in the brain. It was all right there on his monitor. I put a lot of work into that brain, man. It was like seeing a prized car dented.

"Okay, so here's the brain damage," Dr. Kent said, wasting no time. I flinched. When I thought of the term "brain damage," I thought of people who had been permanently incapacitated. I didn't care to think of myself as such. I didn't care to think of my own brain as a tangible object that could be destroyed. How damaged was I, really? After all, I could still see and feel and remember and think.

But I couldn't hear. I looked away from the scan as Dr. Kent told me that I would never hear out of my right ear ever again.

"So there's really no way to bring it back?" I asked him. I knew the answer, but I still held out hope that he'd be like, *Actually, yeah, just eat more fiber and the meatus should be groovy in no time.* But no, he said. The ear was dead. There was no way to resurrect it. Not by natural means, at least.

"Well, that sucks," I told him. I didn't collapse to the floor in despair. I didn't cry. I didn't star in my own impromptu Oscar clip. I just bitched, same way I did when I came out of the coma. I left Dr. Kent's office, got in my Kia, and drove back home. Alone. I was well enough to drive myself anywhere I pleased now, but that was little solace as I sat behind the wheel and took in the impact. Trauma is a vine: a parasitic entity that latches on to a thriving host and, over time, grows on and around it. It can take a while, even years, to make its presence fully known. It doesn't surround you all at once. It just needs time and sunlight, and on my drive home it had both in equal measure.

It got worse. Dr. Kent sent me to an audiologist named Dr. Michael Morikawa, so that they could get a full survey of the wreckage to my internal stereo system. Dr. Morikawa took me into a soundproof booth and tested each of my ears separately, not unlike hearing-test day back in elementary school. He played a distant beeping noise, and I could have sworn I was hearing it through the dead ear. A FUCKING MIRACLE. I told him I'd heard the bad ear spring back to life.

I was wrong. I walked out of the booth and Dr. Morikawa showed me my test scores. For the right ear, I scored a perfect 0.0. I recognized no sound at all with that ear isolated. As a crowning blow, my "good" ear on the left had *also* been damaged. I'd missed out on a lot of high-frequency noises with it. My aggregate hearing capacity was at less than 50 percent. Dr. Morikawa told me that the left ear must have been damaged in the fall. I actually didn't agree with this, because I've spent my entire life with my music turned up to eleven through my headphones, and because my father has a similar kind of high-frequency hearing loss in both ears: a natural by-product of aging. I was due for this shit. But I didn't tell Dr. Morikawa that. I didn't want the insurance company to be like, *Oh, well, if it was inevitable this whole time, let's not cover anything.*

"What about the sound I heard on the right?" I asked him. This is when Dr. Morikawa gave me an impromptu lesson in the biological miracle that is bone conduction. When he'd played a *ping* into my dead ear, it sent vibrations rippling across my skull that my left ear picked up, interpreted as sound, and sent to my brain, which then processed the sound as coming from my right. That is how the brain rewires itself. That is the miracle of biology.

But that meant the apparent resurrection of my right ear was a mirage. I was deaf. And what little I could still hear, I hated.

MIRACLE EAR

Everything was too loud. With only one operational ear, I had less surface area to absorb my kids yelling, ambulances whizzing by, and every other annoying sound the world around me makes on a daily basis. It's the same lesson you learn about weight dispersal in middle school. Imagine someone stepping on your foot with a flat shoe. It hurts, but their weight is spread out over the area of your foot. Now imagine someone doing the same thing, only with a stiletto heel. All of their weight is concentrated on a single, SEXY point, which means your foot will be much, much more aware of the ensuing pain.

This happens with limited hearing as well. You might think that hearing loss would, in a mixed blessing, help blunt the impact of the noise around you. It doesn't work that way. Instead, noises hit with a more forceful impact. My brain, still hardwired to listen to the world in full, was now working double time to organize what little sound it was receiving, which left my hearing fatigued. Vulnerable. It also became much harder to distinguish between *all* sounds, both loud and soft. This is known as the cocktail party effect, and it fucking sucks. For many people who are hearing impaired, the cocktail party effect discourages them from so much as leaving the house. The noise of the outside world is simply too much for them to bear.

I was coming to understand this fear intimately. My first night out after getting hurt was a cocktail party, natch, for my wife's preschool. When I walked into the room, I physically shrank from the ruckus. People came by and said, *Hello, oh, I heard about what happened. That must have been so terrible, but isn't it nice you could come out,* but I couldn't make out many of the words. I sought out bare corners of the room as temporary shelter from the onslaught, self-medicating with mushroom puffs I stacked high onto a tiny plate. Drinking might have helped alleviate the situation, but the last time I'd had a few, it hadn't gone all that well. I was off the sauce for good. I never did have all those Miller Lites I'd asked for in the hospital.

Weeks later, we got invited to a bat mitzvah for Flora's friend, and the cocktail party effect there waged an even more vicious assault. There was an emcee and a band. The emcee was loud, as emcees are paid to be. He took the mic to greet the crowd and damn near blew me out of my fucking chair. I was quietly angry that he was so loud. *Can you believe this asshole screaming at everyone to dance? At a party?* I had to flee to the adjacent barroom. Sonia came out to keep me company.

"Go on back in," I told her. "You shouldn't be stuck out here with me."

"It's okay."

"I gotta find an earplug." I had dozens of earplugs at home, acquired over a lifetime of drugstore visits and business-trip stays at hotels that give them away for free. But I hadn't thought to bring an earplug with me this night. And *one* earplug was all I needed. My right ear was strictly ornamental now. I could have cut it off and worn it around my neck like a warlord if I had felt like it.

By the grace of God, I asked one of the servers and—HEY

PRESTO!—he procured an earplug for me within minutes. This is the advantage of going to any bat mitzvah or wedding or anniversary party. There are always enough old people on hand at these things that earplug demands are commonplace. I stuffed the lone plug into my left ear and finally made it out onto the dance floor.

But the cocktail party effect didn't need mass gatherings to knock me sideways. We lived next to a highway. When Sonia opened the kitchen window—and oh, how she loves her fresh air—the noise from the traffic grated on me. We had lived in this house for a dozen years, and in New York before that. I had long been used to the ambient white noise of traffic outside. No longer. I couldn't stand it. It colored my mood to get pummeled by the Beltway's ruckus, to have it bleed into the regular noises inside our home and render everything a single, indecipherable blur. Whenever two people at the dinner table talked at once, I fumed. And my kids, being kids, talked over each other all the fucking time. Whenever Carter barked suddenly, I jumped out of my chair and yelled, "JESUS CHRIST!" reflexively. I started taking sound breaks, getting up from the table and going upstairs to rest from the noise and to tamp down my frustration. One night I ate my entire dinner in another room because my bad mood had become an environmental contaminant.

Restaurants were their own gauntlet. In the 2010s, the average new restaurant design featured unfinished ceilings, harsh angles, stainless steel everywhere, and a running playlist announcing to everyone that the head chef liked both hip-hop and the Ramones. They *wanted* shitty acoustics. They *wanted* your ears to die while you ate. The trend grew so widespread and obnoxious that servers themselves began to experience permanent hearing loss.

Sonia and I took the kids out for pizza one afternoon after the bat mitzvah. It was your standard Chipotle-esque, upscale-but-not-upscale place where they assemble your pizza in front of you and charge you five bucks more than you wanna pay for it. We got our pies and sat down. Suddenly, the staff turned on the sound system and my ears were under fire. I crammed some pizza down my gullet and fled the premises. I had never taken stock of acoustics when I had eaten out in the past. Now they were all over me. Even worse, I was blaming the source of any noise for making that noise. Real *GET OFF MY LAWN!* shit. My deafness was tormenting me, and putting me at arm's length from both Sonia and the kids. I felt utterly alone inside of it.

I, of course, was not alone. In fact, over sixty thousand Americans become deaf in one ear every year, including celebrities like Brian Wilson, Huey Lewis, and Stephen Colbert. SSD can happen as a result of aging, traumatic injury (that's me), even infection. I never knew this before I lost my hearing. I wish I had. I wish I'd also known that deafness can cause tremendous fatigue. It takes a lot of energy for your single ear to take in so much information over the course of a day, and for your brain to then cognitively arrange that information into discernible sound. My brain, already spent from my rendezvous with death, was overburdened as it was. So by dinnertime every night, my ear was punch-drunk and I was an exhausted, touchy prick. I had my own witching hour between five and six where if something bothered me, I would either seethe or I would let out a "GODDAMMIT" loud enough to stop everyone cold, same way my old man was capable of doing when *he* was pissed. Our mail always came right around then. You do NOT want to open up surprise bills at the end of a workday. When I noticed our bank was charging us illegal fees, I went into my home office to call their customer service and found myself trapped in the automated calling system's maze of twisty little passages. The office door did nothing to muffle my curses.

After dinner that night, Sonia took me into the living room while the kids did their homework.

"You have to cool down," she told me.

"THE BANK FUCKED US."

"So you solve it. Screaming about it won't do anything. The kids hear you, you know. I hear you. It's wearing us all down."

"Yeah, but the bank—"

"No, you. You're different now, Drew. You need to accept it."

"I don't wanna be different."

"But you *are*."

I broke down crying and she took me in her arms. "I can't hear," I told her. "Sonia, I can't hear anything and I fucking hate it."

"Think how far you've come. You can't let this get to you."

It did. Ask anyone who's ever suffered from depression what's the worst thing that you can say to a depressed person, and their reply will probably be "Stop being depressed." I couldn't just will myself to not be bothered by the world doing everyday world things: commuters laying on the horn, kids screaming, banks sucking, etc. I was mourning. Even music had been lost to me. Without two ears, I had lost the binaural effect you get from music, where it feels as if you're hearing it *inside* your mind. I wanted music back. I wanted everything back. In my mind, I had the *right* to be bitter.

But Sonia had the right to not live with that bitterness. The irony was all over me. I am a loud man. Ask anyone. When I talk, I talk way too loud. I like the music and the TV volume way up. Sonia used to beg me to turn the TV down, and I was like, *Sonia, life is loud. Why bother trying to fight it?* To me, loudness was the sound of people being alive and boisterous. It was the commotion I had forever adored to dive headlong into. Trying to contain it was both futile and joyless.

Now I would have given anything to tune that loudness out. I didn't like the noise. I didn't like people talking over me. Sonia had had these same pet peeves all through our marriage, and I had never listened to her complaints. Now, for the sake of our marriage, I had to. It was my turn to understand what it felt like to not be heard. I had to take more sound breaks. I had to recognize when the anger was coming and make the time to go somewhere and quiet it down.

And I had to get hearing aids. If I could make my hearing even a little bit better, it would make the burden of *not* hearing that much easier.

I went back to Dr. Morikawa. He showed me the latest models. I was a potential candidate for two different kinds of hearing aids. The first one was a Baha system, in which an aid is surgically implanted next to the dead ear to amplify bone conduction to the other side of your head. Essentially, this system would amplify the sensation I experienced "hearing" beeps on my right side during my test. The second one was a CROS system, in which you wear a standard-looking aid on the dead ear, which acts as a microphone and wirelessly transmits sound from the bad side over to an aid stationed on the good side, so that the good ear doesn't have to strain to hear what's going on over there.

"You're better off with the CROS," Dr. Morikawa told me.

"Okay."

"Would you be interested in a cochlear implant down the line?"

"I would."

"Okay, well then we can talk about that more later on. But let's get you set up with the aids first."

"Please."

A traditional hearing aid is a strange little device: no bigger than a cashew, with an earmold that fits inside your ear canal. The ones Dr. Morikawa showed me were Bluetooth enabled. OOOOH. I could play Slayer through them, which probably would have damaged my hearing even further, but still!

"Will insurance cover these?" I asked him.

"I'm not sure of that. What we have to do is order yours and then submit the invoice to see if your insurer will cover them. If they don't, we cancel the order."

We had to cancel the order. Hearing aids are not cheap. The ones I picked out cost over $2,000. Per ear. My insurance company explained that they would cover the cost of them, but only through a secondary insurance company of theirs (WHY???) and only using a doctor that the jayvee insurer approved. Dr. Morikawa was not one of them.

But I was still lucky. Insurers rarely cover hearing aids at all, and the result is that millions of Americans don't end up using them. Leaving hearing problems untreated can lead to depression, cognitive decline, and increased risk of dementia. Thanks to the hemorrhage, I was already nut deep in the first two items on that list, and I was a prime candidate for the third. Without the aids, everything I had been suffering through would only get worse until I was stone dead. Not by coincidence, hearing-loss sufferers are also at an increased risk of early death. So if I had to navigate yet another series of quintessentially American healthcare obstacles to get them, and to avoid paying retail price, I would.

I went to a different audiologist named Dr. Lowen. After I went through a whole new cognitive gauntlet to get my records and test results transferred from Dr. Morikawa's office to hers, she programmed a temporary, single hearing aid for my left ear while I waited for a CROS system of my own to arrive in the mail.

"Will insurance cover all of this?" I asked her.

"Yes."

"*Really?*" I'd been hurt before.

"Yes. They'll cover the aids, plus the charger. Now, let me just program the loaner for you." The programming part was important. You can buy hearing aids off Amazon for less than $100. They are, as you might suspect, cheaply made and shitty. But also, hearing aids work best when programmed to accommodate your exact kind of hearing loss. Your prescription, essentially. Correctly programmed hearing aids amplify the frequencies you miss and minimize those your regular ears can still detect, thus keeping outside noise smooth and even. They have settings for special noise situations, restaurants in particular. Using something called a telecoil, they also can connect with sound systems at certain events and broadcast music and/or dialogue straight to your ear. Many theaters and concert halls have signs posted outside indicating that they're compatible with the telecoil, signs I had ignored over my first four decades of existence.

No two hearing-loss patterns are the same. I had a chart from my test with Morikawa, not unlike an EKG, that mapped out the abilities of my left ear in exact detail. I needed a hearing aid that knew my map and could fill in the gaps. Dr. Lowen plugged the aid into her computer and set the program. Twenty-first-century audiology is both a branch of science—though not technically a medical discipline—and a form of IT. Your audiologist needs to have a working knowledge of the hardware involved in treating your hearing loss and the software running on it. They're also there, naturally, to *sell* you that hardware. In America, every discipline of medicine is also a retail outlet. Thus, hearing-aid providers occupy the same mercantile real estate as Warby Parker or your local chiropractor. The sales part tends to be the lead dog.

Dr. Lowen walked around her desk and outfitted the aid on my left ear. The second she turned it on, everything sounded clearer and fuller. I could make out bird chirps coming from beyond her office window. I still had only one working ear, but the boost that ear got from the aid was already evident.

"How's that?" she asked.

"It's actually a bit loud?" I was ashamed to complain. But the levels were off enough for me to hear a doubling effect.

"Lemme adjust it. What about now?"

"Yeah, that works."

"How does it sound when you talk?"

"Lemme see. My name is Drew Magary and I'm wearing a hearing aid. I sound like me!"

"Great. When your CROS system arrives, bring that loaner back, and then we can program your real aids."

"Shit yeah!"

She showed me how to link my aid to my phone, warned me not to let my dog eat the aid, and then sent me on my way. I grabbed some candy from a dish on the front desk and then walked out into a properly amplified world. Cars honking. Doors clapping shut. Trees swaying in the breeze. I kept touching the aid, which produces the same sound as when you rub your fingers on a microphone. A hearing aid is a microphone, after all. Shit, your ear itself is a microphone. It's the greatest microphone ever designed.

Walking to my car, the wind picked up and blew heavily on the mic. Wind is not kind to hearing aids. I was gonna have to get used to that. Also, I wear glasses at night. When you put on glasses, the hearing aid gets in the way and you can hear the ensuing tussle. It's like you're eavesdropping on yourself. But these were minor complaints. I could hear better, and that was all I gave a shit about. Once the proper CROS system arrived, I'd get even more sound dexterously funneled into my left ear. I'd get closer to being myself again.

Getting that system took weeks. Once it did, Dr. Lowen's computer bricked while she was setting the program for both aids at her office.

"Uh-oh."

"What's *uh-oh*?" I asked her.

"It won't let me connect with your system's software anymore."

"Did . . . did you just break my hearing aids?"

"I promise this *never* happens."

Well, it did this time. Dr. Lowen got on the horn with the manufacturer and had to order a whole new system. She assured me I would not be charged for it, since everything was under warranty.

"If you get a bill for these, please let us know and we'll handle it. You shouldn't get a bill."

I got a bill. They handled it.

Meantime, I spent a few more weeks with my loaner. At one point, I took it to Oracle Arena in Oakland (I could fly again!) and found myself by a concourse trash can, changing out the replaceable battery while game 3 of the NBA Finals was going on just a few hundred feet away. The Warriors lost.

Two weeks later, the replacement system arrived. Dr. Lowen fitted the left ear's aid on me and it worked perfectly. Then she fitted the CROS aid onto my right ear. Again, this would not enable my right ear to hear anything. It was there strictly to pick up sound from stage right and tell my left ear about it. But, as with bone conduction, your brain can *interpret* the location of this sound even when it's coming from a secondhand source.

"Can you hear anything coming from that side?"

I snapped my fingers by my right ear. Not only could I hear them snap, but the sound of the snap felt as if it was coming from the center of my head. Already my brain was jury-rigging a binaural effect.

To compensate for my inconvenience, Dr. Lowen's practice gave me a free package of wax guards: tiny, replaceable bits of plastic inside the aid's earmold that protect it from wax, dust, and all the other assorted goodies you ear picks up over the course of a day.

"Can I work out with these on?" I asked Dr. Lowen. I was acting like I had just gotten a free pair of AirPods.

"I mean, you *can*."

"But I shouldn't."

"I wouldn't."

"I won't."

I got in the car and exulted. I was well past the self-consciousness and vanity that accompany the transition into being a Hearing Aid Guy. I was just elated to hear things again. To that end, I blasted the car stereo on the way home. It wasn't perfect, but it was closer to the way I had heard—and sung!—music before the night the lights went out on me. Before this, I had been leaning on old shit for my primary listening: music my brain was already well acquainted with. Nothing too disorienting. Now I could listen to new songs and grasp them.

But I didn't just want to grasp them. I wanted all of them. I wanted my right ear back, and there was a long-shot way of getting it. Seeing that long shot come through would require even more patience, more luck, and perhaps a new hole in my head.

WELCOME TO THE CLUB

My hearing aids were invisible. All hearing aids are designed for maximum discretion. The main receiver of a traditional hearing aid, which houses its battery, microphone, and internal processor, sits comfortably behind your ear. A clear wire from the receiver snakes around your ear's outer rim, or "helix," to reach the earmold sitting inside your ear canal. Your ear canal is a part of your body that people avoid looking at too closely. Same as your feet (if they're ugly), the inside of your nostrils, and the male scrotum. I wore my hearing aids and no one could tell. Whenever I took them off to show them to my friends, they were surprised. It was like I had pulled a quarter out from behind there.

It makes sense for hearing aids to remain hidden, both for aesthetics and as an appeal to the remaining vanity of old folks who are often too proud to wear them. I preferred having mine out of sight as well. The aids were a blessing but also a scar. I wanted all that damage locked away inside an attic. I wanted it erased.

The irony is that the more I was able to conceal my ailments, the more they tore away at my psyche. I didn't need a walker anymore. I wasn't hooked up to an oxygen tank. I didn't have a grappling hook for an arm. No one could tell that anything was wrong with me.

But I knew. And when people can't tell that something is wrong with you, they don't instinctively react to accommodate your discomfort. If you see a hobbled old lady walk onto a crowded subway train, you give her your seat, right? I was not afforded such benefits by strangers. If I walked into a loud-ass restaurant, they weren't like, *Oh, we better turn the music down. The ear guy is here.*

I was disabled. I *am* disabled. My handicapped placard expired shortly after I returned home, but I'm still a member of the fraternity anyway. The old saying is that the disabled are a minority that anyone can join at any time. Halfway through my life, I joined it. So many people are disabled in ways you can't see and perhaps they can't see either.

But now I had my fancy hearing aids. I was all better. Definitely. The day after my aids arrived, I took them off for a moment and told the kids I wouldn't be able to hear anything.

"Oh," said Colin. "You're Deaf Old Dad again."

"That's right," I told him. "Deaf Old Dad. My superpowers are gone for the moment."

I seamlessly incorporated my hearing aids into my morning routine: getting up, grabbing them out of the charger, and nestling them in my waiting ears before hopping onto my phone to see what our asshole president had done THIS time. Every night, I meticulously cleaned the aids like I was an antique toy collector. Meanwhile, my right ear was still nothing more than a tchotchke. The cocktail party effect? Still there. Echolocation? Nope. Still wouldn't know where a truck was coming from if it hit me. The more I recovered from my hemorrhage, the more pronounced my losses became to me. I could deal with the deafness thing. It was all the attendant side effects that came *with* it that were driving me nuts. I continued to be a cranky old turd. You know how old people want to do everything themselves to prove they're still useful, and how they get pissy if you dare infringe upon that pride? That was me. I got angry at people when they failed to speak up loud enough for me to hear. Simultaneously, I didn't care to be defined by what I couldn't do, nor did I want to define myself by it. I wanted it both ways. I wanted to be seen as "normal," but I also wanted everyone to accommodate my predicament without my having to make a fuss about it.

This is the sort of defiance that you constantly see in uplifting movies and in PSAs about anyone suffering from a permanent, crippling malady. But that stubbornness, at least in my case, served as a flimsy cover for outright denial. I knew I was deaf but I didn't *accept* it. I hated it. Whenever people asked me how I was doing and what it was like being deaf, I was like, "Beats being dead!" And yes, of course I was happy I was no longer dead. But on a more practical level, being dead is a breeze. You don't have to fucking do anything. The dead have it easy, and don't let the living tell you otherwise. So I was glad to be alive, but I took that almost as an onerous given. I didn't *want* to spend all day clicking my heels and singing songs about how I'd like to buy the world a Coke. I wanted to not be deaf. I certainly wasn't gonna learn *how* to be a deaf person, even though I could have made that effort and perhaps should have. I didn't want to learn sign language. I didn't want to join a support group. I wanted no part of this new world I had been dropped into. I was being prejudiced against myself, which is a neat trick. This was not how I envisioned my life derailing.

And I *had* envisioned it. All my life, in fact. Well before my accident, I imagined becoming quadriplegic, or being stricken blind, or having my arms blown off by a rocket-propelled grenade while serving in the Special Forces in Kosovo. To say these were daydreams would be INCREDIBLY inappropriate. I didn't want my arms blown off. But sometimes your brain gets antsy, slides a door, and gives you a peek at life in alternate dimensions. There you are, on the losing end of a medieval sword fight. There you are, telling your partner in the homicide unit to go get that damn Mendoza while you lie on the ground, a bullet lodged firmly in your shoulder. There you are, *dead.* In a grave, surrounded by wailing loved ones. I had been through the dying part. Again, not what I had envisioned. Nor had I considered the possibility of waking up one day without my ear. Now it was my reality.

And even if you know that I wear hearing aids, you don't really understand what it's like to have the outside world smothered before it has a chance to reach your brain. Sure, you can plug your ear up to replicate the effect, but you'll always know you can pull that plug out. You'll know it's temporary. The forever component doesn't factor in, and it's a significant one. Also, you can still hear noise through an earplug. It doesn't block out *everything.* Earplugs are not enchanted objects. No matter what stands in a functional human ear's way, it cannot help but do its job. When it can't, there's a laborious process in coming to terms with the fact that you must live the rest of your life knowing you are physically incomplete.

So I told everyone I was half deaf. This was because I have a big mouth, and because I figured they should know about it in advance, in case I missed anything they said. I told all my Deadspin co-workers about it over the Slack app and got a requisite round of "Man, that sucks," which I very much wanted to hear (or, in this case, read). Then I got a DM from my new co-worker Kelsey McKinney.

"I, too, am half deaf."

"Holy shit!"

Kelsey became deaf in her right ear after suffering a cholesteatoma, or inner-ear growth, as a child.

"It ate my hearing bones and eardrum. Very rude."

Kelsey had tried hearing aids and hated them. But she adapted. Rewired. Her left ear picked up the slack and became so attentive as to be superhuman. She also learned, unconsciously, to read lips, not even realizing she could until COVID-19 struck and everyone was suddenly wearing masks. Without seeing people's mouths,

Kelsey discovered she couldn't understand them very well. Nevertheless, she had lived the bulk of her life without a functional left ear and managed to thrive. Now I had a friend in deafness. A one-woman support group that I clearly needed and had refused to seek out on my own. But right away, I felt better talking to someone who had been through my very specific brand of shit.

Sonia, true to form, adapted better to my disability than I did. Whenever she had to tell me something, she made sure she was in the same room as me and that we were face to face. She made sure I got sound breaks both at home and at restaurants. In certain moments, I was less cognizant of my deafness than she was.

She wasn't alone in extending me such courtesies. When I went out to dinner with a friend in LA, I sat to his left without thinking about it. He was facing my dead ear. Even with the aids in, it would still be a challenge to carry on any conversation in that position inside a loud restaurant.

My friend knew which ear of mine was rotten. Without my asking, he switched seats so that he was facing the working ear. People are nice like that. When they know you've got a special need—that's me!—they usually endeavor to make sure you're comfortable. They rewire their own behavior. My indoctrination into the disabled club was something I hadn't wanted, and yet it was proceeding smoothly despite the fact that *I* was arguably the most insensitive one about my condition. I hated who I had become, if only physically. I felt I deserved better, even when people I cared about were going out of their way to help me.

I needed to get the fuck over myself. And fast. But I wouldn't. I wasn't aware of it at the time, but even with the hearing aids in place, I would go on to lose more of my face. Much more of it than I had ever imagined. I guess I should have imagined harder all these years.

NOSEDIVE

Mom and Dad came down to visit in April. They hadn't seen me since I'd left Mount Sinai, and now here I was: upright, well groomed, and encased once more in a healthy amount of subcutaneous fat. My mom's voice quivered when she saw me. My parents are not huge criers. They're not performatively stoic heartland dipshits who think crying is for the weak. They just naturally tend to keep their wilder emotions closer in. The only times I've heard or seen Mom cry were when my grandparents died and when Colin was born five weeks early and he and Sonia managed to survive the caesarian intact. So when Mom so much as chokes up, it's a notable event.

That I had managed to come this far more than qualified as one. I was still shooting for 100 percent recovery, but that's partially because I wasn't awake when doctors drilled holes in my head and gave my family bleak long-term prognoses. I, alone among my family members, couldn't grasp how close I had come to oblivion. I couldn't see it. I couldn't hear it, of course. I was off in fucking dreamland. And I still hadn't summoned the courage to look at the photos of myself comatose. But Mom had seen and heard all of it. That she could see her son now standing up, and that she could hug him, was a goddamn miracle.

"Oh, Drew," she said, "we thought we'd lost you."

"It's all right, Ma. Here I am. Let me help you get your stuff."

"NO, NO, NO! You stay here." She wasn't gonna let me lift a present box out of her trunk. Much too strenuous. Being both considerate and lazy, I didn't push back. She and Dad brought in their luggage, along with the requisite goodies for the kids and a wedge of nice cheese for the grown-ups. To commemorate the occasion, I fired up the smoker and tossed a big-ass pork shoulder on it. Pork shoulder is useful for smoking because it has a wide margin for error. Even when it doesn't fall apart on the bone, it's still a boulder of fatty pork. It's impossible to ruin.

My folks usually brought some wine along when they visited, both as a present and because they like drinking wine. But this time they arrived with no complimentary booze of any sort. I still hadn't had anything to drink since my release. I got mixed signals from doctors about alcohol. One doc from Mount Sinai warned me never to drink again. Another specialist told me to wait at least a year. And another, Dr. Zarroway, said I could resume drinking right away so long as I practiced moderation. I sucked at moderation: with booze, with Cheez Balls, with masturbation, with everything. I didn't trust myself with alcohol, and I didn't want my head to spontaneously combust a second time as a potential result of drinking too much. A brain hemorrhage makes for a hell of an intervention in that way. So I chose to stop drinking entirely. Weed still piqued my interest, but my drinking life died the night of December 5, 2018. Fittingly, I have no memory of my final sip.

More interesting, Mom *also* stopped drinking shortly after I was discharged. She came down with a nasty flu once she got back home. When she recovered, she realized she just didn't want to drink anymore, and that was that. She also wanted to show a bit of solidarity with me, seeing as how I was dry. It's likely no coincidence that my mood routinely swung downward right around happy hour after I got hurt. You build up a lot of edge when you can't take the edge off.

The kids greeted Mom and Dad with gleeful yelps and hugs, mostly because they knew my parents always brought them free shit. My folks also, in one of their trademark bits, offered up enthusiastic running commentary on the kids while the kids were around.

Colin is just a PISTOL. He never stops moving, that one!

Rudy has such a good heart. He refilled my water glass without me even asking him!

You gotta watch out for Flora. She'll outsmart you every chance she gets. Holy shit, nothing gets by that one.

(All true.)

We went for a walk outside. I loved walking with them. I remember the walks I took with Mom and Dad around Manhattan back when I was living there, because Mom insisted on walking everywhere in the city, dragging me block after block like an oversize Colin. I also remember walking with her along Nauset Beach on Cape Cod once, and she walked so far and so fast that I had to tap out and turn around. I remember my dad walking me down a different hospital hallway after I woke up from back surgery in 2006. And of course, I remembered all of our walks together at Mount Sinai. Every day, Mom and Dad helped me out of my bed and walked me to a common room on the other side of the ward. This was basically another patient room, only it didn't have a bed in it. The stroll to that room was better than the room itself. It was my version of going "outside." My walk around the block. I didn't last very long on these adventures, but the fact that I could make them at all provided ample evidence to Mom and Dad that their son wasn't dead just yet. Those walks meant the world to me, too, even if I didn't show it at the time. They reminded me that I was loved and that I was making progress, enough to make me believe that I was finally gonna get out and taste fresh air one day.

So now, after Mom and Dad had walked me around Mount Sinai day after day to nurse me back to health, I got to go on a proper walk with them out in my own neighborhood. Dad has two replacement knees, so he doesn't walk terribly fast. But he never bitches about it. Mom will blaze ahead fifty yards, wait for him to catch up, and then blaze ahead another fifty. They have their system down.

I myself had gotten into walking as a natural by-product of middle age, and because old injuries to my back had put a merciful end to my time as a recreational jogger. When I went on business trips, I walked everywhere in unfamiliar cities, so long as it was less than, say, two miles to get where I was headed. Whenever I wanted to exercise at home but avoid the gym, I walked a five-mile circuit outside that ran along sidewalks, through Metro stations, and across footbridges that spanned the Beltway. Walking was thinking. Walking was seeing. Walking was hearing. Walking was living.

Now I could walk again, alongside two other avid walkers to boot. This was peak spring in the DC area, and few places do spring better. It rains flower petals on you if you stroll through the right places: your own coronation. I saw great swaths of changing colors as we passed freshly blooming cherry blossoms and dog-woods and irises and saucer magnolias. I could hear the flowers lolling in the breeze.

But I couldn't smell them.

If my hearing loss went undetected as a matter of priority, my loss of smell was apparently even lower on the triage list. That's why everything in the hospital tasted down to me. I couldn't smell it. When I smoked the pork shoulder for my folks, I got all of the fat and the salt, but little else.

"Are you guys getting any smoke?" I asked everyone at dinnertime.

"Oh, yeah!" they replied. I was devastated. Smoked foods were the only foods that mattered to me. The first food I ever loved was smoked salmon. When I was in preschool, Mom made me a bagel sandwich with cream cheese and cheap packaged smoked salmon inside for the school's "Lunch Bunch." I remember biting into that bagel the first time and wanting more. MORE MORE MORE. That's how kids grade food. It's not *This needed a bit of crunch, but I like how you married the creaminess of the Philly with the brininess of the Acme salmon trimmings.* It's MORE, PLEASE.

I quickly graduated to other smoked foods: bacon, ham, smoked sausages, smoked trout, whitefish, ribs, pulled pork, smoked *eggs*. I dreamed of one day owning a smokehouse of my own: a charming hickory shack inside of which I could hang salmon fillets and entire pig carcasses. When I bought myself that $250 smoker off Amazon as a Father's Day gift, I cared for it as if it were a preserved copy of the Dead Sea Scrolls. I taught myself how to make every kind of barbecue so that I could have smoked meat on hand anytime I pleased. Now it was gone. Bacon, man. I lost bacon.

After my parents went back home to Connecticut, I tested my olfactory prowess to see what else I had lost. I went to the spice cabinet and held a bottle of vanilla extract so close to my nostrils that I may as well have been picking my nose with it. I barely got anything. I face-dived into a jar of cinnamon. Nothing. I ran upstairs and rummaged through Sonia's perfume supply. I opened a free sample vial and sniffed it at point-blank range. Nothing at all. I couldn't fucking smell. Not even asparagus pee registered.

I had a follow-up appointment with Dr. Kent that week. This was, ostensibly, one of those follow-up appointments that your doctor mandates even though you have nothing new to report and they have nothing new to treat. I was still deaf in my right ear. Dr.

Kent laid out the advantages and risks of having cochlear implant surgery, in which a device is surgically implanted under your scalp, with a series of electrodes threaded through the cochlea, potentially rebooting the dead ear. He mentioned all the potential side effects, including that I could die from the anesthesia, which is a universal surgery risk. It's the Terms of Use fine print you automatically agree to before you register for an Uber account. I blew past that spiel and asked about my nose.

"Smell loss can happen with the kind of injury you suffered. I would add more acid and spiciness to your food to help make up for it."

"Yeah, but is it ever coming back?"

"It could."

"But it also couldn't?"

"That's also possible, yes. The good news is that the nerves that control smell actually have the ability to heal, while other nerves don't. But as you can see"—he brought up my dreaded scan once again, pointing to a vast splotch toward the front of my brain where a splotch shouldn't be—"the damage here was extensive."

I went home and did some research. Up to 25 percent of people who suffer a TBI have their sense of smell affected. It can take years for the sensation to recover, if it ever does. Certain smells might come back but can be initially different from how they originally smelled. A piece of steak might smell like a dog. A toilet might smell like bubble gum. Even though the prospect of this odor dyslexia sounds alarming, it means that something upstairs might be working again, and that your oh-so-clever brain is re-learning which smells are which. One man I spoke to who had also suffered a TBI, a radio show host named Moose, told me his sense of smell came back after *ten years* missing.

For now, my own nose was barren. It's a condition known as anosmia. According to the National Institutes of Health, 3 percent of

Americans suffer from anosmia, and nearly a quarter of Americans over forty have had their sense of smell altered in some significant way. I had been welcomed into yet another club, whose membership went into the millions, that I had never taken notice of before.

The club included my friend Will Leitch, who founded Deadspin and lost his sense of smell when (at least, according to one theory in his family) he contracted scarlet fever when he was five years old. Leitch has no memory of his ability to smell, if he ever had the ability at all. In fact, he has no fucking idea what people are even talking about when they talk about smell. In the beginning, his own father didn't believe that Leitch couldn't smell anything.

"So he started running things that smelled terrible under my nose," Leitch told me, "from dog poop to rotten food, and I had no reaction at all. And then he ran ammonia under my nose, and I started gagging. He was like, *Aha! I knew it! He can smell!* Then he took me to the doctor, and they said, *Don't rub ammonia under your child's nose. That's very bad.*"

I asked Leitch if he ever smelled phantom scents, or if there was a primal instinct inside of him that knew what smell was, even if his brain lacked the ability to process it. But he never had any misplaced smells, and he seemed uninterested in ever trying to reclaim the sense.

"Most of the time people bring up smelling, it's to say that something smells bad. So not only do I not know what I'm missing, I don't understand why it's important. I'm sure if I'd been able to smell at some point, it would matter to me. But it doesn't, because I've never been able to do it."

I wanted to explain to him that smell was *extremely* important, and that he was being way too cavalier about it. But Leitch had no frame of reference to understand the concept of smell at all. So I couldn't tell him that, yes, people call more attention to shit that smells bad because they take good smells for granted. The good smells are the ones you keep between you and your brain. The smell of walking into elementary school on your first day. The smell of a girl's hair when you sweatily hold her close for the first time at a middle school dance. The smell of Popeyes: so thick it feels like they fried your nose.

Smell is ethereal. Yes, in the grand scheme of things, smell is not the top dog. If you had to prioritize your five senses, smell would be dead fucking last every time, even when you factor in what it can do to your sense of taste. But when a smell hits you, it stays with you forever. Like the other four senses, smell has a direct link to your soul. Ah, but how do you even begin to explain how or why it does to someone who's never been able to smell anything at all?

Leitch didn't know what he was missing, and it was impossible for me to explain what the sensation feels like on a physiological level. Certain things must be felt to be understood properly. But let me try to describe smell anyway. Smell is what's in the air. It's your ability to sense, to *feel*, the presence of something that cannot necessarily be seen or heard. And this universe is made of a great many things that you and I cannot detect with the naked eye. Volume-wise, there is roughly fifty-six times more air on earth than there is water. Every day, you wade through an ocean of air that makes the Pacific look like a fucking swimming pool. Your nose is your guide through that unseen layer of existence. If it's not the only way you can sense certain elements of your surroundings, it's often the very first. You smell the fart, and then you see the culprit. Smell is a warning, a welcome, or a mystery that goes forever unsolved. According to a *New York Times* article written by Brooke Jarvis and published in 2021, the human olfactory system contains 100 times more neural receptors than your sense of sight—which is way higher up on the sensory triage list—requires. Jarvis reported that an able-nosed person is able to detect "as many as a trillion smells." Each of them precise, distinct, and memorable.

I wanted Leitch to be more curious. I wanted him to *try* to smell. But people have been getting Leitch to try to smell things—ammonia included—for decades. It makes sense that he would get sick of it.

Besides, thanks to his anosmia, Leitch had superpowers that enabled him to carry out pungent chores that people who can smell typically avoid. As a kid, he was in charge of cleaning out the litter box (the cat's, not his own). As a father, he's in charge of all dead-animal disposal. He also farts with impunity, although all guys do that.

"There's a little part of me that's always still surprised that if I have a quiet fart in a car, people find out about it really quickly," he said.

So Leitch knew how to live without smell. I didn't, and I didn't want to. I had good incentive to reclaim my powers. Smell dysfunction can lead to a loss of appetite, other poor eating habits, and depression. Even worse, getting smell dysfunction treated here in America is exactly as fruitless an endeavor as our healthcare system would lead you to expect. It's almost always viewed as a symptom of a greater problem—which I very much had—and not a root problem to treat on its own. Loss of smell is also now infamous for being a potential symptom of coronavirus, which means maybe I got coronavirus two years before everyone else did. I was into coronavirus before you even heard its first album.

All Dr. Kent could suggest for me was that I take some zinc. The zinc did nothing. In April, my neuro-rehab doctor, Dr. Zarroway, told me that the only place in the entire country that prioritizes research of anosmia is the Monell Center, which is loosely affiliated with Children's Hospital of Philadelphia. No shortage of smells to examine closely in that city. I emailed the center to ask for help. Monell was flooded with inquiries from COVID victims during the pandemic. But in 2019, they weren't nearly as deluged, which is presumably why one of the doctors there was able to write back to me right away:

> *The olfactory nerves are particularly vulnerable to damage because they pass through a bony plate on the way to the brain. The force of a blow to the head may cause them to be pushed against that bone and crushed or severed; injury to the more central olfactory regions is also possible.*
>
> *Unfortunately, there is no established treatment available for such damage. The olfactory system is resilient, however, with neurons in both the olfactory bulb and epithelium being continually replaced throughout the life span. Thus, there is the potential for spontaneous recovery (the best estimates suggest that 30–40% experience recovery of smell following head injury–related loss, although estimates vary wildly), but it is typically delayed and gradual, often taking two or more years. While recovering, many patients develop dysosmia (distortions in odor quality perception) and/or phantom smell sensations. There's no compelling evidence that zinc supplementation is beneficial for smell loss.*

I had yet to reach the dysosmia phase of recovery, if I would ever reach it at all. But even though the Monell Center couldn't offer a proven treatment for my condition, the doctor there told me that there was one thing I could do to give my nose a chance.

SMELL THERAPY

onell referred me to Chrissi Kelly, a British smell researcher who has suffered from anosmia since 2012 and heads up a foundation called AbScent (see what they did there), which is dedicated to both raising awareness of smell loss and finding a cure for it. You can go to the AbScent website and test your snout to determine what exact kind of smell loss you have and why you have it. I filled out their questionnaire.

How did you lose your sense of smell?

I answered, "brain injury."

Do you sometimes smell things that other people can't smell, like something burning?

I did not.

Can you sometimes recognise some sort of smell, but don't know what it is?

I could not.

Can you tell the difference between salt water, sugar water, and water with a little white vinegar in it?

To answer this, I ran to my kitchen and downed a spoonful of every option. I did *not* dilute the white vinegar. Ever have a teaspoon of vinegar? Don't. It tastes like a teacher in 1908 is punishing you for saying the Lord's name in vain.

The good news was I could taste all of the required flavors: sweet, salty, and acidic. I got my test results back:

You may have TBI (traumatic brain injury) anosmia. You do not have phantosmia. You may have parosmia. Your sense of taste is ok.

I was elated to read this, even though I knew it was only a half-truth. Yeah, I could taste the basics. But smell is a critical factor in distinct flavors, such as bacon. Smell some bacon with me now. Lay some strips in a pan. Hear them sizzle. Watch them shrink and curl. Let the heady aroma of salt and hickory flow up through your open nostrils. You can already taste the bacon in your mind. Smell not only informs flavor but also the *anticipation* of flavor, just as sight and sound and touch do. Comedian Artie Lange once wrote that the best thing about cocaine was going to get it. Bacon ain't much different. Without any sense of smell, I had lost a critical delivery agent of that anticipation. I had also lost the smokiness, although that has yet to stop me from partaking when a tray of fresh bacon is within eyeshot. The fancier your food is, the more smell factors in. Smell is what gives certain foods nuance that you can spend years learning to recognize and understand. Now I had lost that nuance, demoted to having the palate of a middle-school kid. I went out into the yard and grabbed a sprig of mint to chomp down on. The menthol in it lit up my tongue, but the inherent mintiness of the leaves was gone. I tried some mint chocolate chip ice cream. It was just chocolate chip ice cream now.

Beyond food, I mourned the loss of smells I might never experience again. The smell of a baby's head. The smell of chimneys piping out smoke late in the fall. The smell of the ocean beckoning you as you get closer to the beach but can't see it just yet. The smell of pizza sitting in the passenger seat after you pick it up. The smell of sex, which is funky in a way that is deeply alluring on a primal level. You get every possible body fluid commingling down there, and you stop pretending that bad smells are a turnoff. You stop holding back everything in your mind and body. That's when sex gets good and *nasty*.

I missed farts, too. You might think it's a blessing to live life without smelling farts and to have your shit literally not stink. You are dead wrong. While I now possessed the ability to use a porta-potty without fear, I missed the more everyday flavors of shit smelling. I could crop-dust Sonia and the kids all I liked—and I still do—but I couldn't bask in the damage I'd wrought because I couldn't smell it. Tragic. The only smell I *didn't* miss was barf. That was about it. The smell of vomit has made me vomit *again* far too many times for it to engender happy memories.

There was also the crucial functionality of being able to detect bad smells. If there was a fire or a gas leak, I wouldn't know. If food went bad, my nose wouldn't be able to clue me in. When Will Leitch was in high school, he breached a gas line with a post-hole digger. Because he couldn't smell jack shit, he thought he'd struck an air line. The way you fix an air line is by—you guessed it—lighting a match to melt the plastic piping and seal it shut. The only reason Leitch is still alive right now is because he couldn't find a match that day.

Thankfully, Sonia could smell milk gone wrong from eight counties away, but left on my own I'd be in danger of unwittingly eating leftover taco meat infested with botfly eggs. Sonia left a hunk of feta in the fridge one day and I crumbled a small hunk of it into an omelet. After I finished eating, she walked into the kitchen and gave the cheese a sniff.

"OH GOD, THAT'S GONE BAD!"

"Uh-oh."

Somehow I didn't die of salmonella. And hey, at least some of that feta didn't go to waste. But for reasons both practical and personal, I needed to get my smell back if I could. To do so, AbScent recommended smell training. I bought two smell kits off of their website: one for me and one for my old man (who had lost his sense of smell thanks, again, to the ravages of age). My smell kit contained four jars, each one housing a cotton disk soaked in an essential oil. The separate odors were clove, rose, lemon, and eucalyptus. These are the primary colors of scent. You can make your own smell kit, but it requires going to the local health food store and buying tiny bottles of rose oil tincture. I was too lazy to do that. The sales copy from AbScent read:

> These jars are more suitable for beginners because they offer the "smelliest" experience.

That was me. I was a beginner and I wanted the smelliest experience. I threw down £23.99 (plus shipping) and eagerly awaited my maiden voyage into smell therapy.

My smell kit arrived in the mail. It came with instructions. Yes, I laughed at that the same way you're laughing right now. Who needs instructions to smell? Well, I did. I had to find a quiet place to sit. No distractions. I had to uncap each jar, one by one, and hold it to my nose for thirty seconds at a time. And then I had to think about what I could smell in the jar. Not what I was *supposed* to smell, only what I could physically detect. If I couldn't smell anything, or if I could smell only part of something, that was okay. The kit also included a little worksheet, so that I could record the strength of each scent (I never did this).

"Try to explore the smell in as many ways as you can," the pamphlet instructed me. So I did. I held the clove jar to my nose and got a distant trace of Thanksgivings past. A fresh pumpkin pie coming out of the oven, waiting to be topped with whipped cream. I moved on to the rose jar and got a tragically weak reminder of the spring unfolding right outside my door. I barely got anything from it. But I got *something*. I wasn't all the way gone. I treasured whatever tiny smatterings I could detect.

Clove and rose were the hard smells. The AP smells. Every session, I made a point of doing those jars first and saving the other two for last. Eucalyptus was the strongest. It's a sister scent to mint, only more aggressive, which served my purposes nicely. I was a happy little koala bear, huffing eucalyptus and feeling it clean out my sinuses. Was that a smell? Or was that feel all I was getting? I wasn't sure, but I figured that feeling an odor had its own value. Indeed, when I cooked dinner that night, I leaned in to the tomato sauce heating up on the stove and took a big fucking whiff. I felt *something*, only to realize that it was just the inside of my nostrils getting really hot. Felt good, like I was taking my nose to a Russian bathhouse. I wagered my brain could use that information constructively.

Lemon was my dessert smell. It was the oil I could detect best, and also, the smell of lemon is a happy smell. It's fresh and bracing. I could have smelled lemon for more than thirty seconds a pop, and I did. The AbScent copy suggested I visualize a lemon while I was sniffing the lemon jar. No trouble there.

Even so, smell therapy wasn't easy. I was still stuck on what I couldn't smell and not on what I still could. That nose-half-empty attitude wasn't doing me any good. Second, I still had terminal internet brain, which made it hard for me to focus on anything for thirty seconds at a time, least of all smells that barely registered. I got impatient just waiting to finish EXHALING before I could sniff again. Like millions of other people, my attention span had been destroyed. It was like that long before I suffered my brain hemorrhage. Thus, I rarely reserved time in my life to sit there and concentrate on a single sense and that sense only. The exception came whenever I ate. When I eat, I don't want anything coming between me and my compromised bacon.

Otherwise, gross impatience rendered my other sensory experiences mere wallpaper. When's the last time you smelled something and just smelled it? How often have you literally stopped and smelled the roses? Before I got hurt, I think I focused on a smell maybe twice a day, maximum.

Now I had to force myself to smell and smell only. Smelling is its own form of meditation. The AbScent pamphlet included the same phrases that you hear listening to a session on the Calm app. "It's easy to get distracted. . . . This is normal and happens a lot." "You should feel confident this is something you can do with practice." "Try not to judge."

I tried not to judge. Like I said, I genuinely missed all smells, good and horrible. To that end, I expanded my smell training to outside the kit. I took heavy sniffs of cut-up fruit and thought hard about what registered. I smelled Colin's hair. He wasn't a baby anymore, but the nape of his neck still had that unmistakable kid musk to it. Little bit sweaty. Little bit powdery. Whenever I hugged him, I took in as much of him as I could. If I saw any other big smell nearby, I rushed to claim it.

That included Carter. He was far removed from his last bath and the kids, adhering to a ritual they had practiced ever since we adopted him, smelled his fetid body and went "EWWW-WWW!" in unison, begging Sonia to give him a bath (Carter was not in agreement with this request). I joined in on the group whiff, hoping to get a scintilla of dirty dog. It's a reassuring stench. You smell your dog, and you know he's a dog. I didn't get much, but I felt Carter's fur tickle my nose, and that was its own reward.

I took Carter for a walk and he paused to take a dump by the side of the street. I picked up the turd and, making sure no one was around, buried my nose in the bag to see if I could catch anything. I recoiled, but only a little bit. There was *something* distressing in the air. If I hadn't known I was inhaling my own dog's shit particles, I'm not sure I could have placed the smell. Also, who's to say I wasn't simply imagining a smell being there when there wasn't one? I wasn't above tricking myself.

My sense of smell had become a missing child. I was waiting for it to return, and feverishly latching on to any sign of hope that it might. I kept huffing my smell-kit jars. I once inadvertently smelled one so hard that I sucked the disk up from the jar to my nose. Sometimes I worried my own exhalations *into* the jar would somehow taint the oil inside. Sometimes I sniffed too hard and snarfed a booger into my throat.

But on I sniffed. I sniffed sweaty clothes of mine that had been fermenting in the laundry basket. I sniffed fresh bread. I tried to sniff more farts, waving them into my nose like I had nasal Munchausen syndrome. I stepped in dogshit—which usually never fails to enrage me—and seized upon it as a chance to experiment. I got nothing. I sucked on a lemon, Thom Yorke style, to see if I could get the full lemon experience. It had zip out the ass, although my tongue was almost certainly doing all of the grunt work.

The calendar flipped to May. I went to the gym and thought I smelled something in the locker room. Something clean and soapy. I went to the sink area and sniffed around like a bloodhound. I'm sure this looked very normal to the other gym members. I lathered my hands up with enough soap foam to wash down an old Pontiac, and then I planted my face in the suds. Nothing. It would not be the last time I thought my smell had walked back through my front door.

Sonia and the kids forgot about my situation well before I did. They'd be like, "You smell that?" to the room, and I'd point to my nose, rolling my eyes, to remind them. My hearing loss was a noticeable matter to them. My loss of smell, less so. Just as Leitch couldn't comprehend having smell, everyone else can't comprehend *not* having it. Even if you plug your nose and walk around for five minutes, it ain't the same. You're just making a librarian voice as a temporary goof. There's no existential crisis at hand.

But I was stuck on the prospect of never being able to smell important things again. My memories of smell were slipping away. If you have a fully armed and operational nose, it's impossible to forget smells because you can just smell them again to get a quick reminder. But when you can't, your memory is all you can bank on. I could still remember certain distant events like they were yesterday—my first kiss, the day I split my head open at Mitch's apartment, my wedding day, 9/11. But even though smell and memory are inextricably linked, it's very hard to recover a smell on its own, even if you have the right visual memory on hand to goose it. My smell history was evaporating, consigned to eternal invisibility.

The scent in the smell jars grew so faint that I became concerned that the oil on the disks had lost their musk altogether. I called the kids over to sniff the eucalyptus jar, and it nearly knocked them over. Nope. The disks still worked.

"You're lucky your smell doesn't work," Flora told me. She and Leitch should go bowling together sometime.

"You'd think this was a happy development, girl. But it's not."

"Yes it is." Given her age, Flora was not terribly open to persuasion. In her defense, if you can still smell, it *does* sound nice to never have to smell dead skunks or hot garbage or bad cologne ever again. But it's a superficial blessing, because those smells are indelible. They're important, just like all the good smells that you definitely notice but often keep to yourself.

Eucalyptus, for instance. Eucalyptus is one of the main ingredients in Vicks BabyRub, which Sonia and I used on all the kids when they were infants. BabyRub was a gentler version of Vapo-Rub. Whenever baby Flora got a cough or a stuffy nose, we laid her down on the changing table before bedtime, took a little swipe of BabyRub, and massaged it into her chest to clear her throat and sinuses. We sometimes did this in the middle of the night, when Flora was awake and fussy right when neither Sonia nor I wanted her to be awake and fussy. These were the sleepless nights every prospective parent is warned about, and they are the forge in which new parents are made and hardened.

The BabyRub was a refuge on those nights. I remember the scent vividly. Smelled like some medieval doctor had whipped up an herbal remedy using a mortar and pestle. I remember being *excited* to give Flora the rub. Rudy and Colin, too. When it's 3:30 A.M., it's just you and your kid. Alone. In the dark. You can't see. You can only hear, touch, feel, and smell. The bad sensations dominate: loud crying, smelly barf, diapers fully saturated with acrid baby piss, the baby inadvertently ripping out your chest hair, etc. Of course, now that my kids were older, I *missed* the smell of their spit-up, just as I missed the better, more intimate scents from those late nights. I missed hearing them coo. I missed being able to rest their heads—the whole head!—inside the crook of my elbow. I missed the BabyRub. I missed eucalyptus. When I got those faint traces of it from the jar, I got to time-travel back to those nights.

Memory can be kind in that way. It'll safeguard the good parts of your history, and then it'll spit-polish (or outright reengineer) the bad parts. But when I lost my smell, the retouched memories that came packaged with them became harder and harder to reach.

And there was no guarantee that those memories would ever fully awaken once more.

We had a glider for the nursery when our kids were little. We got our money's worth out of it. It was white (bad idea) with colorful little dots all over it, like a slice of Funfetti cake. Over the years, that glider accumulated a layer of baby-barf stains that turned the base white upholstery into more of an eggshell color. A Barfetti cake. We gave the glider away. That's how the cycle works. You accept that you no longer have use for your baby gear because your kids aren't babies anymore, then you pass it on to other parents who are a few miles behind you on the road. I miss that glider. I remember sitting in the glider and I see the stains, I hear the crying, I smell the spit-up, I feel my children squirming and clapping in my tired lap. I'm glad I had all my senses for those times. They might turn out to be some of the final fully sensory experiences of my existence. Not a bad way to go out.

Because the sum total of everything your senses take in is what makes a *feeling*. Every sensation I experienced in that glider is connected within a single, critical memory. As time passes, the memory is all you're left with. I don't mean that in a sad way. Memories are a gift, even the shitty ones. They're the files you have on hand in your mind to go back and see and hear and touch things that you may no longer be able to see and hear and touch. I'm glad my kids are old enough where I never gotta listen to the fucking Wiggles again. But I also *miss* the times they liked the Wiggles, just as I miss the smell of applying a little eucalyptus rub onto their ailing bodies. Those feelings are life. They're you. They're everything.

But I was growing tired of locking myself inside my home office to concentrate on smells that were barely there. This wasn't an existential brand of dread. Not this time. I was just getting bored with the process. I brought my jars out to the TV room and did all my smell therapy while watching basketball. The AbScent pamphlet specifically said to NOT do this. But my focus and my determination were both waning.

Clearly, I needed more stimulation. I went hunting for it in the form of bureaucratic vengeance.

SUE YOU, SUE EVERYBODY

Technically, I was at a work party when I got hurt. Univision, which owned Deadspin at the time, was footing the bill at the karaoke lounge. The awards show itself was a promotional vehicle for Deadspin, even if it prominently featured a demo toilet onstage. But was I *working* working? According to Univision's lawyers, I was not. While I was comatose, Sonia filed a workers' comp claim with the state of New York. Faceless entities from both Univision and my insurance company—and a strange solar system of tertiary insurance companies working in tandem *with* my insurance company—moved to deny my claims, blaming my injury on drinking too much (their estimation). I appealed, calling the New York State workers' comp board. I filled out more forms than a law school applicant.

My appeals were denied. The fact that I was claiming workers' comp in New York despite not actually living in New York only made the board's bureaucracy more ornery. Also, workers' comp tends to be reserved for those who have been injured as a direct consequence of the physical work of their respective jobs. If you're a construction worker and a steel beam lands on you, you got hurt because of your job. But in my case, doctors didn't know why I had collapsed. And because they didn't know, the amorphous blob of lawyers opposing my case said that there was no definitive proof that my work that night could be blamed for it. Maybe I would have collapsed at home. Maybe I was like someone working at an office suffering a heart attack at their desk. You can't prove that work caused that heart attack, unless you happen to be working at Amazon. Sonia was convinced my work that night factored into the accident somehow, but neither her hunches nor mine counted as admissible evidence.

Still, despite the fact that I had been cleared to return to work full time, I had lost my ear and my nose. We had also paid thousands of dollars in medical bills, thanks to all the neat loopholes in the American healthcare system that allow insurance companies to leave a seemingly random portion of expenses your responsibility. If I had any shot at recovering that money, I needed to take it, despite the fact that I had since returned to work at full capacity and the fact that workers' comp is really meant to compensate those who can't. I didn't grasp this. Here is where I could go for cheap self-deprecation and tell you this is because I'm an idiot, but I'm not. I'm a demonstrably smart man, and so my ignorance about workers' comp was more a form of gruff denial.

And perhaps avarice. I ogled New York's Schedule Loss of Use chart, which assigns set values to specific work-related injuries. For example, if you lose an arm, you're entitled to a maximum of 312 weeks of pay for the loss. A hand? 244 weeks. A big toe? 38 weeks. The schedule I checked on the state's website noted that loss of hearing also merited an SLU award, but it didn't say how much. I wanted to know.

Loss of smell, as you might have guessed, didn't appear anywhere on the chart.

I requested a hearing. New York lets you attend these hearings remotely via video call: a convenience that would become all too necessary nationwide in 2020. The board said I didn't need a lawyer for my hearing. I asked the union in charge of Deadspin if they could grant me a lawyer anyway. They said I had to hire one myself. I believed, with genuine idiocy this time, that I could handle the case on my own. I demanded SATISFACTION, and blithely assumed that my accident spoke for itself. To that end, I wrote down a list of arguments to make in front of the judge. In my mind, my virtual hearing would take place inside a formal courtroom, complete with a stenographer and perhaps even a ragtag jury of my peers. I needed to be both persuasive and stately. So I prepared my case. It consisted of a one-page document in Microsoft Word.

Your Honor . . .

- Please note that I do not live in New York and that my accident occurred while I was traveling for business. I ought to be covered for that entire trip. I do not believe I would have suffered this injury under normal circumstances at home.

- Also, opposing counsel claims I was *not* "performing a work-related activity." This isn't quite accurate. I was out at a lounge with all of my co-workers, my boss included, in a casual setting, which could easily count as team building. We were there to celebrate the awards show we put on, and likely to break it down after it just happened. To say it was a "purely personal and recreational activity" makes it sound like I was not with my colleagues. I would not have been at that lounge nor with my colleagues had I not been "within the scope of my employment." And to say that my employer "derived no benefit" from me going to the function is debatable. We were building camaraderie. No, it was not at a traditional work site, but it was a work function. Two of my co-workers told me Univision paid the tab at that function. If it wasn't a work-related activity, why was it on the company dime?

- The statement from counsel says that I hadn't eaten that night. This is untrue. I had pizza at the lounge. Victor brought it.

- There is nothing in medical reports explicitly stating that my injury was caused by alcohol, which means that counsel cannot prove an "injury has been solely occasioned by intoxication from alcohol."

- Also, I submitted medical records to the board showing that I have permanently lost hearing in my right ear as a result of the accident. I believe I am entitled to compensation for this schedule loss of use.

I rehearsed these bullet points again and again, reading the words out loud and tweaking them for maximum vigor. I had been inside courtrooms in the past, for jury duty, for speeding tickets, and for my own DUI arraignment back in 2009. I already knew that a real courtroom is nothing like *To Kill a Mockingbird*. If you make a touching closing argument that serves as a damning indictment of both the prosecution and AMERICA, they fine you $500 for holding up the line. No matter. In my heart, I knew I had an airtight case. And if I knew this, surely everyone else within the legal system would understand.

They did not. I called up opposing counsel before my hearing (this is something that's legal to do) to go through what to expect during the hearing and to ask him, straight up, for advice on how to win.

"Do you have a lawyer?" he asked me.

"No. Does it matter?"

"Your odds'll be better if you have a lawyer. But given that you have no documented proof that hosting the show is what caused your fall, those odds are still fairly slim." He wasn't trying to intimidate me. This was a credibly nice lawyer I was talking to. Besides, my case was a wart on his firm's ass. Whether or not I actually won it didn't matter much to him either way.

I wore a suit for the videoconference. The judge let me in from his office. He was NOT wearing a robe. He was dressed like a normal, everyday white-collar worker. Also in on the call was opposing counsel: a woman sitting at an empty conference room table, staring down at some template script her firm had used a million times for all such proceedings.

"Mr. Magary, do you have a lawyer?"

"No, Your Honor. I'm representing myself."

"Okay, I'm gonna dismiss your case right now because I don't see much cause for it to go forward. Now, keep in mind you can appeal for another hearing, but I strongly recommend you retain counsel if you wish to move ahead with it."

Just like that, it was over. I expected my hearing to be a full trial for some reason. It was not a trial. It was formal paperwork shuffling. Nobody has time to hear a fucking sermon during these things. But I hadn't diligently typed up all of those stunning bullet-point items just to have them go unread. If I told the judge all of my grievances, maybe he would go bug-eyed and summarily reverse his prior decision.

"Your Honor, can I just make a few points before we end this call?"

"Of course."

I fired off my arguments.

"I completely understand where you're coming from," said the judge, starting to sound like a customer service operator. "That's why you'll want a lawyer if you want to continue moving forward with this." I got his formal Notice of Decision in the mail days later, citing "insufficient medical evidence" to advance my case. The letter had a typo in it.

I called lawyers. One of them explained to me that it was foolish to pursue a workers' comp claim when I had already returned to work full time, with no hindrances going forward. I had been filing forms up the wrong tree.

"Can I just, like, sue Univision in general then?"

"Possibly. Your case is actually quite complicated, because you don't live here and you were at a work party when you got hurt, not at work itself. But send me all of your medical records and other relevant information, and I can make a better evaluation."

I sent the lawyer all my files. He never called back, not even when I called his office multiple times to poke him (now that I think about it, perhaps calling him so much had the opposite effect of what I originally intended). I called another lawyer and got one of what sounded like many, many assistants. I had reached his processing center. I sent them my files as well. Nothing. Across Manhattan and Queens, there are file boxes sitting in unoccupied legal office closets as we speak, containing sensitive papers outlining the story, and the cost, of my brain going SPLAT. I imagine these papers burning a hole in each box, as if they were the cursed insides of the Ark of the Covenant. In reality, they'll remain buried alive until an incinerator comes calling.

One lawyer finally called me back. I was sitting in a parking lot when Lazlo Oswald (that's not his real name; I have given him the best imaginary Bronx lawyer name I can think of) called me and told me that my case compelled him.

"Really?" I asked.

"Yes, I think there's something here," he said, in an unidentifiable Eastern European accent. "Now, what's important is that you remember everything you possibly can about that night in the bar. Is it possible you slipped on a spilled drink?"

I didn't see how that factored into my case against a gigantic media conglomerate.

"I really don't remember," I told him. "I don't remember anything."

"Is it possible anyone saw you slip and fall on this drink?" he asked me. The spilled drink was a given to him now.

"No, sir. No one saw me fall." The only person who had "seen" it happen was Jorge Corona, who had seen only its immediate aftermath. Univision security had already conducted phone interviews with Jorge, Sonia, Megan Greenwell, and my other colleagues about the night in question, all for the sake of an internal workers' comp investigation.

"Because they have very hard floors there," Mr. Oswald said, continuing to lead me. "So if a server spilled a drink and you slipped on it, they're potentially liable."

"Wait a minute," I told the guy. "Are you talking about suing the *bar*?"

"Yes."

"But I was talking about my potential case against my company."

"In my opinion, you have a much better case against the bar."

"I'm not sure I wanna sue the bar."

"You're not really suing the bar," Mr. Oswald told me. "You're suing the insurance company. All these restaurants and bars have coverage for this sort of thing. So we could potentially extract millions of dollars from the insurer without putting the bar out of business."

Suddenly, I wasn't feeling so guilty about the idea. Millions of dollars *and* we could stick it to BIG INSURANCE? Sounded like a strong play all around. I felt I deserved some sort of recompense for what had happened. Someone needed to pay for this; if not God, then a similarly faceless, omnipotent entity. Preferably one with deep pockets.

I also knew that whenever you find yourself in either insurance hell or legal hell, you are alone. No one else gives a shit. The system is designed to leave you feeling helpless, lonely, and, ultimately, unmotivated. Mr. Oswald appeared to give a shit. It was the *wrong* shit to give, but he was the only person working within the hell industrial complex who appeared genuinely interested in what happened to me.

"All right, Mr. Oswald, what are the next steps?"

"The next steps are you remembering everything you can."

"I told you: I remember nothing. I blacked out."

"Well, think hard. It could come back to you. Maybe you saw a puddle on the floor, you know? Maybe you remember your legs slipping out from underneath you. You're gonna have to testify to that for this to work." He wanted me to lie. "So will you think on it and then get back to me?"

"Uh, okay."

"Great."

We ended the call and I got out of the car to do my errands. I tried to remember the specifics of my accident while grabbing a bottle of Coke Zero and a beef stick. Doctors told me memories of that night could, conceivably, return to my consciousness after lying dormant for a long period. Physical trauma, like mental trauma, can be actively suppressed by your brain in the interest of protecting you.

But I had nothing. I pictured myself slipping. On a concrete floor. While wearing hiking shoes I had changed into after the ceremony was over. I visualized the "accident" a few more times, one of those strange instances where if you insist upon a false memory, it has the potential to become very real to you. But it wasn't real to me. I don't know why I collapsed, but I did know it wasn't because of something like *that*. I also knew I wasn't gonna lie on the stand. I couldn't. I suck at lying even worse than I suck at moderation.

I drove home and never called Mr. Oswald back. There would be no massive payday. No legal vindication after I had somehow been wronged by a bar that dared to have a floor. I never sued. When I called the bar for this book and left a message, no one called back. They also never returned any of my emails. Soon thereafter, in the midst of the pandemic, the bar closed. Their phone number now gets you the dreaded special information tone. You know the one. *Doo-doo-DOO!!!* at 400 decibels. That one. The bar's website domain is now available for anyone to buy. I did not buy it.

I never appealed a final time for workers' comp. At the end of May 2019, I received one last letter from the board, along with a check. Apparently, the insurance company that handled workers' comp requests on behalf of Univision had failed to file a "notice of controversy" (in legalese, "controversy" means the formal raising of a dispute, not that I slept with Kate Winslet) in a timely manner. Thus, they owed me a penalty. That penalty? $300. That's what my ear and my nose were worth to the system.

All I would get after that was what I already had. Existentially, that was enough. I had been told so over and over again. I said it to people myself. "Hey, I can't complain!" I lightly joked to them. But really, I felt like I wasn't *allowed* to complain. I felt like I had lost the right to be unhappy about things that sucked.

That didn't stop me from trying to exercise that right anyway.

VOICES IN MY HEAD

"There are a lot more 'goddammits' at dinner," Sonia told me. "I'm sorry."

"Flora pulled me aside the other night and said she's afraid to talk to you at dinner because you might get mad about something."

It was true. Even though six months had passed since I had gotten out of the hospital, I was still an overly sensitive prick. Even worse, I didn't like being *told* I was being overly sensitive. Maybe everyone else was being *in*sensitive to the guy with brain damage, I thought.

They weren't. Sonia and the kids were just treating me normally, the way I specifically hoped they would. I repaid them by periodically lashing out. I took basic comments as passive aggression. I smacked a whole lot of countertops. When anyone in the house remarked about a smell in the air, I would testily shoot back, "Well, I wouldn't know about it," reminding them of my anosmia. When my family didn't like something I'd made for dinner, I fumed. My fits had become a matter of routine. Colin told me, point blank, that he liked pre-injury dad better. So did I. I didn't like this new fella I'd become—didn't even know who he was—and I was hoping everyone around me would help compensate by showering me with constant praise and affection.

"You know, the kids see you," Sonia told me. "They're learning to be like this."

"Let me be pissed for *one* goddamn minute! Christ!"

"It's more than a minute."

I cared about Sonia's opinion more than anyone else's, which also made me overreact to it whenever it was negative. I wanted nothing but positive feedback, which isn't how any decent marriage works. You exist to keep each other's bullshit at an acceptable level. I wasn't holding up my end of the bargain. I was too busy screaming about how the world was deliberately making my life more difficult. I spent so much time yelling at customer service reps on the phone that Colin covered his ears anytime the mail came late in the afternoon. If someone barged into my office when I was working, I made a stink face at the interruption. One time Colin came in while I was in the middle of something and I gave him a *What the fuck do you want?* look that was so nasty, he physically recoiled. He feared my reaction. He feared *me*.

When I was a kid, I feared my old man's wrath. Dad never smacked me or anything like that. And he didn't yell a lot. But when he did yell, he made it count. He got *pissed*. I didn't want Dad pissed. I wanted everything back the way it was before Dad got pissed. Then Sonia and I had kids of our own, and I expected Flora, Rudy, and Colin to all fear my ire the way I had feared Dad's. I expected them to fall in line when I got mad. After all, I was just as loud as Dad and twice as profane. But Flora *never* fell in line when I got mad. She straight up laughed in my face every time, even when she was just, like, four. And I'd say to Sonia, "These kids, man . . . They don't fear us! It sucks!"

Without fear in the arsenal, I felt like we had no ability to control our kids, even though I'd read and nodded along with every single modern parenting guide and progressive dadding take. Hell, I'd *written* some of those takes: yelling is a waste of time, lecturing

your kids only encourages them to tune you out, use positive reinforcement more often than negative reinforcement, etc. But I still
counted on fear as a useful fire extinguisher to keep under the sink.

Well, now my kids feared me. That they told Sonia this outright was the clearest sign. Kids never give up the goods like that
normally. I had failed. I wasn't delighted to possess an emotional
shock collar for my kids. I was gutted, the realization slowly creep-
ing into the center of my mind, like the ghostly sound of a cello
playing all alone atop a barren hill. I had become an unpleasant
man. There was a reason, after all, that the dreaded Larry had requested to be moved to his own hospital room when he and I were
forced to share one. It wasn't because he was the asshole. It's because *I* was. He wanted to get away from me more than I wanted
to get away from him.

If you've ever lived with a TBI survivor, or you are one yourself, my case is probably all too familiar to you. According to the
National Institutes of Health, over half of TBI sufferers experience
mood swings and clinical depression, often for life, after being injured. Lemme put on my lab coat for a moment and explain the
physiological reasons for this.

Your brain has three parts: the cerebrum, the cerebellum, and
the brain stem. It's protected by the dura mater, a hardy membrane
that lies between the skull and the brain. The cerebellum, which
is in charge of movement, is a little walnut tucked underneath
the cerebrum. The brain stem acts as the exit ramp to the spinal
cord, sending out instructions from your brain to the rest of your
body. The brain stem controls most of your involuntary body functions: heartbeat, blood temperature regulation, perspiration, etc.
In medical-community parlance, it's your reptile brain. When I
collapsed, I fractured my skull in not just one but three places: the
temporal bone behind my right ear, the frontal bone close to my
left eye, and then the occipital bone, located at the back. My skull

was a real pinball that night. A blood vessel inside my dura mater exploded from the impact, hence a *sub*dural hematoma.

Technically I had *also* suffered a stroke, because a brain hemorrhage is a type of stroke. A stroke is, in the words of Dr. David Heller, "any insult to the blood vessels of the brain." I love hearing the word "insult" used in a clinical sense. So my hemorrhage was a stroke, albeit far less recognized as such compared to a blood clot in the brain: the more common type of stroke that had affected virtually everyone else in my recovery ward at the hospital. Two years after my accident, many people my age would suffer those brain clots after contracting COVID-19, and would do so within the confines of Mount Sinai, the very hospital where my own life nearly ended.

Normally, your brain is protected by four ventricles, or cavities. Unlike the heart's four ventricles, which are filled with blood, the brain's ventricles are filled with cerebrospinal fluid, which provides a layer of cushioning between brain parts. On the night of December 5, 2018, my growing subdural hematoma caused an "almost complete compression," according to my file, of the fourth ventricle separating my cerebellum and my brain stem, leaving both intensely vulnerable. That's why Dr. Caridi had to crack my skull open. He had to drill past it so that he could drain the leaking blood, thereby releasing pressure and giving my brain stem room to breathe. If he had failed, I would have suffered an uncal herniation, in which the brain stem is forcibly displaced. I had herniated disks in my back three times and lived. I had also suffered a hernia in my scrotum. Again, I lived. Not terribly comfortably, but I lived. But you cannot herniate your brain stem and live. You will not be able to breathe if that happens. This is why the brain stem is located *deep* inside your head, at the center of the dance floor. It's the skeleton key. It has to be protected at all costs.

Dr. Caridi and his team at Mount Sinai succeeded in protecting mine. Wildly. They had achieved the most favorable outcome. My initial prognosis said I would "take months to recover from this but may recover faster if the eye movement problems are purely due to peripheral CN8 [cranial nerve #8] damage and not due to central brainstem damage." And indeed, my very mild eyesight problems went away after just a few weeks of rehab. Doctors had saved my brain stem, which meant that my body could get on with the day-to-day business of living, in accordance with the most optimistic forecast they could envision.

My cerebrum was a different story. Thanks to the additional impact I suffered in the front of my head, my cerebrum was—*is*—damaged for life. The cerebrum is home to what you typically think of as your mind: emotions, memories, cognitive skills, etc. It's the boss of your head. You can solve trigonometry equations because of your cerebrum. You can remember the first time you got laid because of your cerebrum. You are dismayed by shitty tweets because of your cerebrum. It's the big part of your brain: the hemispheric sponge you visualize anytime someone says the word "brain" to you.

The cerebrum has its own geography to account for. In my case, the parts of my cerebrum that housed my intellect, my command of English, and my ability to solve basic problems (how to clean up spilled milk, etc.) were left miraculously intact. Other parts of it were not so fortunate. My temporal lobe, which suffered the brunt of the impact, is home to neurons in charge of both memory and hearing. While my long-term memory was preserved, there obviously remains a two-week gap in there that, much to Lazlo Oswald's chagrin, I will likely never recover. That lobe is also in charge of hearing, which, again, is not in good shape.

My smell? Well I could *see* the loss of smell on Dr. Kent's monitor, in the form of white spots around my frontal lobe: the largest part of your cerebrum and one that controls smell, personality characteristics, and other vital functions. Just under that lobe is the olfactory bulb, which sounds like one of those syringes Sonia and I used to suck boogers out of the kids when they were toddlers. The olfactory bulb is not a syringe. It sits on top of your sinus cavity and acts as customs agent for smells to reach the frontal lobe, the piriform cortex, and the thalamus, the last of which processes those smells into rose petals and shampoo lather and fresh cupcakes for your enjoyment. If I'm lucky, the main cause of my anosmia was damage to CN1 (cranial nerve #1), which can potentially be recovered. But there is also the grim, and likely, possibility that the damage to the front of my brain has rendered the recovery of that nerve a moot point, leaving it with nowhere to bring smells after the olfactory bulb has rubber-stamped them.

I'm speaking in uncertainties here, but that's not because I failed to do my homework. It's because the brain itself is a wild and uncertain beast. By the time you read this book, doctors will know more about the brain's physiology than they did while I was writing it. They will never finish learning about the brain, just as we, as a species, will never have outer space fully mapped out and explored. There is too much to know. That's thrilling from a research standpoint. Imagine delving into a subject that has a nearly inexhaustible supply of new things to discover. It's like Columbus never existed. But when it's *your* brain that's the never-ending source of mystery, well, then that excitement gets tempered a wee bit.

Not only was my brain its own little house of mysteries, but how I had injured it remained elusive. I had never fainted before in my life. Sonia believed that the Z-Pak, the booze, and the adrenaline from hosting a small-scale awards show all somehow conspired to bring me down. If that were the case, I feel like any talk show host would have had a dozen of these hemorrhages by now. None of the possibilities presented to me were all that credible. Doctors couldn't even ascertain whether or not my hemorrhage caused my collapse or vice versa. Chicken or the egg. Everyone wanted to know why my brain exploded. They'd put on their deerstalker hats and fire up their pipes and speculate aloud that this mystery *must* be solved. THE GAME IS AFOOT. But all of their attempts to solve it had turned up fallow.

As for me, I knew the answer might hold the key to making sure I didn't suffer another goddamn hemorrhage. Maybe I had a heart problem that hospital EKGs hadn't been able to detect. Maybe God struck me down because I was a shitty gift wrapper. Maybe all my years of drinking really had come back to haunt me somehow. That one doctor who told Sonia that I was exhibiting symptoms of alcohol withdrawal? I have to consider that they were right. Or maybe my days playing football had finally caught up with me . . . twenty-one years after quitting the sport. I smashed the back, the side, *and* the front of my head that night. The reason for the impacts and their sequencing remains unknown. As Dr. David Heller told me over the phone, "I cannot understand it. I feel like none of the doctors explained the physical mechanism whereby this happened to you."

They didn't. They couldn't. Only an ambulance came for me that night. No one ever filed a police report. Maybe my head hit the floor and then ricocheted off the wall, and then back against the floor. Maybe vice versa. Maybe I *had* been assaulted; beaten to near death in ten seconds by either the fastest assailant in the world or merely the luckiest. Whatever happened, it can't be undone. The fact that I suffered a hemorrhage is doubly irritating because "hemorrhage" is a word that I never, ever spell right on the first pass. It's an impossible word. I will have to spell-check this book seventy-five times after it's done to make sure I didn't fuck it up. Up until I suffered one, I only thought of "Hemorrhage" as a fine butt-rock song for karaoke. Now the word would be affixed to me for the rest of time.

The brain damage resulting from that hemorrhage included scars on the front of my brain that will never heal. Here's something that is not a mystery: The frontal cortex, which is located in the cerebrum's cockpit, has a big say in your emotional response to things. When you get shitfaced and moon a parade route, that's because alcohol impaired your frontal cortex's judgment, which is *your* judgment. The frontal cortex, according to researchers affiliated with McGill University and the Canadian Institutes of Health Research, also controls the levers that tell other parts of your brain to dispense the organic chemicals—serotonin, for instance—that regulate your mood. So when your frontal cortex gets a little owie, it's gonna have an effect on that mood. I know this because I used to always cry out "FUCK!" and smack a wall anytime I bumped my head on anything: low doorways, tree branches, or the trunk hatch of our minivan, the last of which seems strategically designed to injure the cranium of any tall person.

So when you permanently damage your frontal cortex, as I did, it can permanently alter your mood accordingly. Since my hemorrhage, I haven't accidentally bumped my head against anything. (Finds largest possible piece of wood to knock on; knocks on it.) This is due to equal parts luck and vigilance. I'm always keeping an eye out for those sharp corners, you know. But I didn't need to walk into a plate-glass window to have my frontal cortex go off anymore. It was forever off. And the worst part was that I couldn't perceive it. I wanted to be fine and, within my mind, I *was* fine. But you can feel fine and still very much not be. The National Institutes of Health sums up the conundrum TBI recovery poses thusly: "Individuals are challenged by deficits of which, in some cases, they are only partially aware."

This was ironic because I spent the bulk of my adulthood preaching self-awareness to people. All around me, I saw dickheads acting like dickheads because they didn't know they were being dickheads. I talked to my friends and to my kids and even to fucking college audiences about it. I told them that self-awareness was the key to being a happy and tolerable human being: to know why you're doing what you're doing and to be clinical in your assessment of yourself.

But that was inaccurate. Being self-aware is an easy gateway to becoming self-centered, and I was certainly self-centered both before my accident and after it. Not only that, but being self-aware gives you license to do the wrong thing even when you know you're doing it. Admission is permission. I used to say to everyone, "I think I probably drink too much," and then what did I go do? Drink too much. Self-awareness is you saying to other people, "Tell me my flaws are pretty." I had lost my right to that convenient form of self-awareness in the fall, and all of the cheap excuses that came with it. I needed Sonia to say, *Hey, man, you're being an asshole,* for me to realize I was being an asshole. It was the only way to know the truth. And I had to *agree* with that truth. I couldn't just paper everything over in "sorrys" and expect it to work. "Sorry" is the most overused, empty word in the English language. It's a word people use to avoid all of the work that goes into absolution. Nothing more.

I said sorry to Sonia a lot. It was worthless. She said as much. Your spouse teaches you how to be a spouse. Your kids teach you how to be a parent. If you fail to listen to them, you'll fail to become the best possible version of yourself. I could blame my brain damage for my irascible personality all I liked, but I *was* my brain damage. I had to go by what Sonia and the kids told me, and what they told me was that I needed help. There was no need to sort out which parts of me had been affected by brain damage and which parts of me were, frankly, just always annoying. After all, I smacked counters and yelled at banks plenty before I got hurt. I was no rookie. There was something inside me that had always needed fixing. The hemorrhage only made it all the more glaring.

I went to Dr. Zarroway again and told him about my problem. I downplayed it to him. "I'm a bit crankier," I told him. "I don't hit anybody or anything"—this part was true—"but it's definitely noticeable, the crankiness." He prescribed counseling for me, plus Keppra: a drug that is nominally used to prevent seizures but has also been used more recently to treat mood disorders, even though mood swings are a listed potential side effect of that very same drug. In America, the cure usually is the disease.

Keppra was the secondary option. I was supposed to get counseling first, then go on the meds if the counseling proved ineffective. I called around. No counselors who took insurance were available near me. Ever. One counselor I called had an opening, only to retract the offer once they realized that I needed to be treated for personality changes brought on by a head injury. They weren't qualified to do *that* sort of counseling. I applied to be part of a study at Mount Sinai to examine emotional responses in TBI patients. If I qualified, I would get to participate in group therapy sessions twice a week, with the results going back to the hospital and to the NIH to help future recovering TBI patients. I filled out yet another form. They screened me over the phone and asked me a series of questions about my current condition.

"Do you hear voices in your head?"

"No."

"Do you think the TV is trying to send secret messages to you?"

"No."

"Do you ever want to harm yourself or do you ever have suicidal thoughts?"

"No and no."

I didn't qualify for the study. I got $10 for doing the screening, though. Despite harboring a longstanding fear of antidepressants—*what if I lose my edge?!*—I took the Keppra. Two days into the prescription, I asked Sonia if she noticed any difference.

"You're better," she said. Not all the way better, she clarified, but better relative to the dickhead who had been stalking around the house of late, ranting and raving about his needy brain. That man didn't want to even play with his own children late in the day. He didn't like going out. He dreaded talking to people. You could chalk that up to him growing older, but lots of old people are happy to see other people. Happens all the time in line at the Safeway.

I didn't want to be this person. I wanted to be who I was, and I remained deluded that I could. The more I tried to be that Other Drew, the more frustrated I became. I had to give in. I had to understand that my injury had not only changed me but also changed everyone I loved. I needed to understand that my best bet for salvation was embracing the very people I was keeping at arm's length. "My job is to translate the world for you," Sonia told me. "That's what marriage is all about." But I kept hoping that medication and time would render that translation—along with therapy and honest self-criticism—unnecessary. I lacked the brainpower to see how foolhardy, and how selfish, that plan was.

But, in a stroke of drive-by luck, the bureaucracy that had proven so indifferent during my little Johnnie Cochran phase was about to turn in my favor. Something was coming on the horizon. Something that would render Sonia's translation of the world much clearer to me. And louder.

THE IMPLANT

I took it as a given that I would never be eligible for a cochlear implant: a relatively new piece of technology in which a surgical device is fastened to your skull, attached to the cochlear nerve, and assumes all of the aural labor that a destroyed inner ear was once able to handle. The most famous recipient of cochlear implants is the late Rush Limbaugh, who had his severe hearing loss corrected when doctors attached implants to both sides of his rotund head. Limbaugh swore by these implants, and it's the first and only time I've ever trusted that man's opinion on *anything*.

Limbaugh could afford these surgeries, but most people can't. They run upward of $100,000 apiece (that's more than my craniotomy cost), and insurance rarely covers them. This was especially true in my case, because the FDA had yet to approve cochlear implants for anyone suffering from single-sided deafness. The reasoning was that if you could hear out of one ear, it wasn't a medically urgent matter to restore hearing in the other.

Dr. Morikawa, working in tandem with Dr. Kent, told me that there had still been a few instances in which insurers covered SSD implants anyway. The fact that I had already gotten my hearing aids covered was, shockingly, irrelevant to my insurer's potential decision.

"So they might cover my implant?" I asked Dr. Morikawa.

"Possibly. The way we find out is we schedule the surgery, and then we wait to see if your insurer will approve it."

"They won't approve it without us scheduling it first?"

"Correct. Do you want to move forward?"

"HELL FUCKING YEAH I DO, DOC."

I picked a date in August and waited for my insurance company to give me the formal stiffarm. Bad news from doctors or insurance companies can arrive in so many different guises: a terse form letter, a garbled voicemail, a vaguely worded email that's harder to parse than a Supreme Court decision. I was ready for all of them. Ready to be crushed. I even thought briefly about how or if I could pay for the surgery myself if it came to that. *Maybe we can take out a loan.* I told friends that I was due for surgery but that it would probably be canceled at any moment. I'm a Minnesota Vikings fan, after all. I'm good at fatalism. Every day we got closer to the surgery date, the more I braced myself for rejection.

The rejection never came. In fact, in a stunning bit of serendipity, the FDA approved the very implant that I had chosen—from a company called MED-EL—for SSD patients two weeks before my surgery date. A week later, I got a call from my insurer saying that my surgery had been formally approved.

"Are you sure?" I asked the operator. I was flabbergasted.

"Yes, sir."

"All of it? Even the equipment?"

"Yes."

I gave her the insurance codes for the surgery and for the equipment (I had to look all the codes up) to make certain that what she was saying was covered was actually covered. I simply didn't believe her. I thought she was granting me approval for just the consult, or the pain meds, or a fucking post-op Band-Aid or something. But no. No, she meant the whole thing.

"Are you DOUBLE sure?"

"Yes, because you fulfilled the rest of your deductible earlier this year." If I hadn't fulfilled the deductible, this wouldn't have been the case. I imagined potential injuries I would have inflicted upon myself to reach that deductible in order to get full implant coverage. Luckily(?), my physical rehab had already eaten all that money up. Insurance makes no fucking sense to me and never will. But that didn't matter now. My right ear was gonna come back. The FDA had bailed my ass out with the play clock running down.

I was given strict hygiene instructions for the night before surgery. I had to shower vigorously using antibacterial soap. I couldn't find any body wash in the house with an explicit "kills bacteria" claim on the label, so I rushed to the store and grabbed a bottle of Dial for Men Odor Armor wash: the kind of male-targeted cologne soap that comes in a gunmetal-gray bottle shaped like the controls of a fighter jet. I took a shower and scrubbed every pore and crevice clean of lethal microbes, snuffing them out with sandalwood-fragranced precision. I bet I would have liked how I smelled. But when I stepped out of the shower and dried off, Sonia took one whiff of my musky freshness and recoiled.

"Oh my God, no."

She relegated the new, manly body wash to Rudy and Colin's bathroom.

I couldn't eat before surgery. I also couldn't drink water after midnight, lest I turn into a gremlin on the spot. I got up the next morning and brushed my teeth, careful to not swallow any Colgate lather. I followed all of the written instructions to the letter, but worried about other, unwritten protocols I might have missed. *Should I put lotion on my face? What about deodorant? Will Speed Stick somehow leach into the incision and fill my ear with chalky aluminum?*

I put on the deodorant.

Sonia drove me to Georgetown Hospital. We parked on the street outside because the "valet" parking cost a hefty seven bucks.

The hospital made us arrive at 5:30 A.M. for a 7:30 A.M. procedure, like we were going through customs at Dulles for a flight to Beijing. I had no say in the surgery time, only the date. Given how nervous I still was about insurance actually covering the implant, I was loath to call the hospital and be like, *Umm, yeah, that's a little early on our end. Mind if we bump that to around ten-ish?* And since I wasn't allowed to eat that morning, I *wanted* them to cut me open at oh dark thirty so that I could eat sooner rather than later.

We got to the hospital's reception desk and they handed us a slip with a number on it, like we were waiting in line at the DMV. I couldn't sit. Too antsy. Instead, I paced the hallways and used the bathroom once, twice, three times to calm my nerves. Along the walls I saw framed pictures of various wild animals: giraffes, zebras, king penguins, hammerkops, elephants, and more. I was certain that someone in the psych ward of the hospital had conducted a study proving that these pictures helped soften the angst of patients about to be wheeled into an operating room. I was also certain that this study's findings were *correct,* because I enjoyed looking at a still of a rhino lapping up water from a cool spring running across the savannah. Soon it would be ME getting to enjoy some fresh water action. I just had to undergo another major head surgery first.

Posted next to the reception desk was a one-sheet document outlining every patient's rights and responsibilities. One of the responsibilities listed was "to meet financial commitments."

I went back to staring at the rhino.

A nurse came out from behind the desk, stepping over and around all the other ailing patients who were splayed out on the waiting room chairs and desperate to find a comfortable position. Looking around any hospital waiting room is always a useful reminder that there's someone there who is worse off than you are. My family learned this firsthand while I was laid up at Mount Sinai. Now I was getting a taste of it. In this case, I had been

DREAMING of getting this surgery. When I'd told people earlier in the week that I was going under the knife, they gasped with
concern. And I was like, *No, no, no, this is good, I swear.* This was
the Good Witch surgery.

The nurse found Sonia and me. I was on deck. She led us to
the back. I always feel like a VIP getting out of a hospital waiting
room. BYE LOSERS! WE'RE GONNA GO HANG WITH
THE COOL PEOPLE NOW! We got to a large bullpen of
gurneys—each one cordoned off with a tasteful curtain—where I
was told to strip down. That included removing my underwear "for
sterility purposes." Seemed like *not* having my balls out would be
the cleaner way to go for everyone involved. And, as you've already
read, comatose Drew was bad at keeping his genitals to himself.
But alas. After getting naked, I had to put on the requisite assless
hospital gown: the one scientifically designed to rob you of your
dignity. But I was used to this ritual now. I was good at being one
of many bodies crowded inside a hospital.

The nurse gave me slipper socks and a hairnet, the latter so that
I could dish out sloppy joes to eighth graders in a school lunchroom
later on. Dr. Scott, the attending, stepped through the curtain to
get me ready. I had read a shitload about cochlear implants prior to
my surgery. I traded emails with patients who had gotten them. I
even talked to a dude who got two implants and then went to work
for one of the manufacturers. I read testimonials for the surgery
like I was scrolling through Yelp reviews of a neighborhood Buf-
falo Wild Wings. And yet here is the question I asked the doctor
right off the bat: "So, you don't drill into my skull for this, right?"

"Actually," said Dr. Scott, "we do, yeah."

"Oh."

"We bore a small hole next to your ear and then thread part of
the receiver through it."

"I knew that."

"I have to put an IV in you."

If you're a connoisseur of getting poked with needles, as I now am, you know that getting an IV is one of those routine pricks that can be more painful and involved than it seems at first glance. I pride myself on having nice, veiny arms. As a bonus, my skin is so pasty that you can see, with your naked eye, many blood vessels available for the injecting of things. I would make a FANTASTIC heroin addict. Dr. Scott knotted a rubber tourniquet around my arm, tearing out vital arm hair as he went. He asked me to make a fist and then dug the needle in.

"Nuts," he said under his breath. "Blew it out."

Blew it out?

He tried again. Another vein blew out. I began to wonder exactly how many veins I possessed. Finally, the designated anesthesiologist sauntered in (they're always so relaxed, like they're high on their own supply) and commandeered the needle. He gave me the usual, legally mandated disclaimer that general anesthesia could kill me, and made me sign forms to indicate that I had been made aware of this. I signed them quickly, like I was paying for Chinese takeout.

I was the first scheduled surgery of the morning for the ENT team. You don't wanna be the last one on the docket: the final obstacle between your surgeon and a bottle of cabernet waiting for them at home. I wanted my team of surgeons *fresh*. Alert. Pumped and jacked to cut my noggin open.

They still made me wait an extra half an hour.

I was not conscious when I was taken into my emergency craniotomy. But for this surgery, I was. Trumpets blared in my mind when the nurses told me it was finally cuttin' time. They wheeled me into the operating room: lights shining brighter than the house lights at Irving Plaza. The surgery team was ready for my arrival, freshly scrubbed and prepped. There was gonna be a blood party and I was the guest of honor! WHEE!

The anesthesiologist returned, rolling up to my side on his stool, as kindly anesthesiologists are wont to do. He injected a new vial of serum into my IV.

"Is that gonna put me under?" I asked.

"Yup."

"Okay, that's cool. I wonder how long it taaaaaaaaaaaaaaaaaaaaa-aaaaaaaaaa . . ."

I was gone. Another dreamless sleep. Another gentle preview of death. When I woke up, I was in the recovery area with a fresh bandage wrapped around my poor, battered head. Even though my right ear had been rendered deaf eight months earlier, it still *felt* things. It very much felt that operation. I was not gifted a coma to dodge the pain this time around. I felt a dull ache deep inside my ear, like a kid had been using my eardrum for band practice while I was out. The outer ear itself grew full, which is not an uncommon sensation when you have ear damage. When I turned my head, I felt a rising thrum on the right side of it. It built to a crescendo and then slowly ebbed. A lot of people who suffer from hearing damage experience tinnitus or some other form of internal sound torture. I was lucky enough to avoid tinnitus after my hemorrhage, but now I was getting a temporary taste of it. You don't want tinnitus. Wear some earplugs the next time you go see Cannibal Corpse live in concert.

Also, my nose was bleeding. I was told this was normal. You're told everything is normal when you're at a hospital. *That arrow sticking out of your back? We see that all the time.* I jammed a roll of gauze up my nostril, which kept my nose from barging in on my ear's big day.

Like an unruly child, I felt around the side of my head even though I had been ordered to leave it alone. There was a hard cup under the bandages, keeping the tender ear safe. I ran my fingers along the gauze, hoping to strike a bump in my hairline. I found it. For weeks afterward, I had friends touch the bump for kicks. They were into it, or at least they acted like they were. Who *doesn't* love touching a weird protrusion on a forty-two-year-old man's head, I ask you?

Sonia handed me a granola bar and some water, both of which I consumed more carefully than I had anticipated. Surgery, after all, doesn't give you a hefty appetite. It doesn't give you much in the way of energy, either. This was an outpatient procedure. *A procedure,* I had told myself on the ride to the hospital. Not a surgery. Totally different thing. Even after everything I had been through, I still approached convalescence like a game I could *win*. I was better at sudoku—studies show that puzzles can help keep looming dementia at bay—now than I ever had been pre-accident. Ear surgery? It was NOTHING to a man with such "high cognitive reserve," as my postcoma neuropsych evaluation had declared. I had actually planned on working that afternoon.

One turn of my head in the recovery room and I was quickly disabused of that cockiness. I was not gonna be able to work that day. I was gonna nap and then cradle a warm cup of tea in my hands like it was a newborn puppy.

I nibbled on the granola bar and realized that I couldn't taste much of it. Nothing salty. Nothing sweet. All I got was the soft, pliable texture of the bar. Parts of your taste are controlled by CN7 (cranial nerve #7), or the facial nerve, which runs through the inner ear on its way down to your mouth. This nerve can get dinged during cochlear implant surgery. Mine got dinged.

Dr. Kent, who performed the operation, came by my bed with a coterie of nurses and protégés to check on me. This is always a nice moment after a successful surgery, when the docs return to you with broad smiles and cheerful prognoses. You're the star again. My surgery was a success. This hadn't been a guarantee. Dr. Kent wasn't going to be able to ascertain the full extent of the damage to my inner ear until he was *inside* of it. There was a chance that a cochlear implant would not be able to bypass that wreckage.

It could and it did. Dr. Kent told me that Dr. Morikawa had

come into the OR while I was under to test the implant and that it was receiving signals perfectly.

"I can't taste anything," I told Dr. Kent.

"Yes, yes," he said, nodding quickly. "That can happen, but it will go away."

"Oh. Okay."

Sonia drove me home. I had to keep my wound wrapped in the bandages for at least two nights, and I couldn't shower until those two nights were up, either. No musky shower gels for me.

I tried sleeping that first night with the bandages on, and it was miserable. I yearned for the anesthesiologist to roll up to my bed at home and shoot me full of triple propofol to put me down. But he, along with proper REM sleep, was nowhere to be found. I was warned to not attempt lying down on the side of the incision. Awake in the dark and bored to death, the first grader in me couldn't resist seeing what would happen.

The nurses were right to warn me. Just thinking about turning to my right was enough to piss the dead ear off. The ear's sensitivity makes it an attractive bull's-eye for sadists and masochists alike. As post-op pain goes, mine was fairly light. But one turn in bed offered me a taste of what a vengeful eardrum was willing to inflict upon me. I feared what it would do if I sneezed. In a small miracle, I wouldn't sneeze for *eleven days* after surgery.

I stayed flat on my back that night and prayed for daylight to hurry. Much to Sonia's chagrin, I still tossed and turned. Bereft of the ability to roll onto one side and then the other, like a poorly cooked rotisserie chicken, I scratched my face at least ninety thousand times. Sonia elbowed me to get me to stop.

The next morning, feeling closer to myself, I violated doctors' orders and pulled off the bandages. Pulling off bandages is now my thing. I carefully loosened the gauze and pulled it away from my head, hoping it wouldn't take my right ear off with it. This time, my impetuousness didn't cost me. Dr. Kent's work was impeccable. The wound was already healed, which was stunning because underneath the gauze was no protective cup of any sort. It was all dried blood that I had been knocking on. I succumbed to temptation, grabbed a Q-tip (you're already gritting your teeth), and gingerly felt around my ear with it. I pulled the Q-tip out and the ear fired yet another painful warning shot across my synapses. Never, ever use a Q-tip after ear surgery. You're not even supposed to use them in your ears at all.

I felt along my new scar and tugged, ever so gently, on the now-loose ends of the tape suture holding my skin together behind it. I looked in the mirror and saw a mutant. My right ear was reaching out from my head like it wanted to pick an apple from a tree. I hadn't considered how a cochlear implant might change my looks. I knew there would be a bump. I knew I would have to stick a magnetized sound processor on the outside of my head and walk around looking like Lobot from *Star Wars*. But now my precious facial symmetry—which many competing modeling agencies assured me was *flawless*—had been disrupted.

I stupidly thought this look might be permanent, until I googled "ear sticking out cochlear implant surgery" and was reminded that all surgeries produce something known as "temporary swelling." And now you know it, too. You are welcome. The swelling was so pronounced that it ended up spreading the temples of my glasses, and I don't even wear glasses during the day. This was why I was going to have to wait another month for Dr. Morikawa to turn the implant on. The swelling had to go down for the processor to stick, and it wouldn't do so on command. To quicken the healing process, I stuck a cooling eye mask—the kind of thing you buy at Brookstone as a thoughtless Christmas gift—in the fridge and soothed my ear with it.

I snapped a reverse selfie in the bathroom mirror so that I could get a better view of the incision. The skin around it was yellowed and badly bruised. Sunlight came beaming through the antihelix of my outer ear—the flappy cartilage part—but a purple contusion spreading across it blocked out the light in ominous patches. I got into the shower, again violating protocol, and washed the hospital off me from the neck down.

We drove to the beach. My family had already planned this vacation before my surgery was scheduled. When the hospital came back to me with a date and time, I figured I could thread the needle and make it work somehow.

"We don't have to go to the beach," Sonia told me.

"No, no, no," I insisted. "We'll go and we'll have FUN!"

Before the surgery, I had asked Dr. Scott if I could go swimming in the ocean with my ear still healing. Doctors are very good at giving measured, calm replies to requests that are plainly ludicrous. In between blowing out all my blood vessels, he told me, "Afraid not."

Fair enough. We went to the beach anyway.

I was under orders to keep my wound out of the sun, so I bought a nylon sun hat with a floppy brim that wrapped all the way around. A true dad hat. I looked like an old college football coach observing two-a-days from a golf cart. Once we got to Dewey Beach, I spent the entire week frolicking up to my knees in the water (Sonia was vigilant, dinging me whenever I tried to wade in any farther). Before dinner every night, I walked three blocks from our house to smoke cheap weed nuggets next to a dumpster behind a Quality Inn. The dumpster had a fence around it, so it was the perfect place for me to pack my fake cigarette pipe and take puffs without anyone witnessing the crime. I spent those little smoke breaks praying a garbage truck wouldn't come by at that exact moment to empty the dumpster and drop it back down on my head.

I didn't drink or toke up for six months after my hemorrhage. You get older and you live in streaks: X number of months without drinking, X number of years since your last prostate exam, forty days without red meat, etc. My drinking streak remains intact. By the time this book is published, it will have been thirty-four months since my last beer. Weed was another matter. I asked a doctor friend if weed also needed to stay off the table forever. Her (fake) name is Dr. Lucien, and I called her directly because I was paranoid about asking her about weed in a text.

"Okay, so I found that weed could actually be beneficial to your recovery."

She wasn't lying. Many retired NFL players, like Hall of Famer Calvin Johnson, not only use marijuana as a safer way to treat their own brain injuries, but have also sponsored ventures into researching the benefits of medical marijuana for victims of chronic traumatic encephalopathy. One of those studies, currently being conducted at Harvard, was endorsed by the late professor Dr. Lester Grinspoon, the founding editor of *The American Psychiatric Association Annual Review* and *Harvard Mental Health Letter*. These studies have not been spurred by mere hunches. According to the *Chicago Tribune*, an *Oxford Academic* study showed that lab mice that were given cannabis after suffering a TBI recovered their cognitive functions faster and better than mice that were *not* given cannabis. So not only were the stoned mice healthier as a result, but they got to be stoned too. Imagine being a stoned mouse. Think of all the cheese you could eat.

When Dr. Lucien gave me the green light, I was quietly relieved. I had been a good and sober little boy, but holy shit, did I need a release. I asked Sonia for her blessing. "Please," she said. The first time I got high post-hemorrhage, I became as calm as a reservoir. Sonia looked at me and said, "You need to smoke that shit every day. Like at four P.M."

I did *not* smoke up every day, and I swore off taking weed candy from strangers ever again. But I did get "jolly" (our code word for it) when the occasion suited me, like while recovering from ear surgery at the beach. The weed was most fine. Also, my little hiding spot was far enough away from the house that no one nearby could smell it. I was far more cautious about masking my weed than I had been about protecting my brain for over four decades. Very predictable of me.

One day, I took the kids fishing at Lewes pier. We bought a bucket of minnows for bait. It would be the only fish we'd encounter that morning. When I grabbed one of the squiggly minnows out of the bucket to bait a hook for Rudy, I gave it a whiff. The minnow stank. It absolutely fucking stank. I put my nose to the bucket and reveled in the bouquet. Whatever smelling power I had left could identify these minnows. I'm certain I was the only person on the pier that day that enjoyed the smell of dying fish. We brought the bucket home and I kept sniffing it, because I could still smell nothing else.

That night at the beach, we went to Funland, a boardwalk amusement park chock-full of Russian kids working summer jobs and trashass Eagles fans driving in from Philly. Near the ticket booth, I spotted a bald man walking by wearing a sound processor behind his right ear. He was in the implant club. *OMG, he's one of us.* I was so, so close to stopping that man and asking him a million questions. *Sir, I couldn't help but notice you have a cochlear implant. I have the implant, too! They haven't turned it on yet! What's it like when they do it? Does it work? Can we be ear friends?*

I did not stop him. We did not become ear friends. The guy was small but could have easily beaten my ass. Instead, I bought Colin a shark tooth necklace and then we all rode the Sea Dragon. My first amusement park ride since my accident. I did not ask my doctors if I was allowed to ride a giant ship that swings like a pendulum higher and higher until your wallet falls out of your pocket and down to the ground. I trusted what precious instincts I had left. Those instincts served me well. I rode the Sea Dragon once, twice, three times. I'd earned the thrill.

But I still couldn't taste a fucking thing.

TASTELESS

The next day at the beach, it rained. Bereft of sunlight, our only entertainment options for the day were to stay at the house and watch shitty TV or venture out to a series of nearby outlet stores. Given the weather, those stores promised to be more crowded than Penn Station at rush hour.

We chose the outlet shopping anyway. You would have too if the alternative was playing sad games of Uno and staring out the window wondering why God had forsaken you.

We were in an Adidas outlet store. Rudy and Colin were looking for new shorts because (a) they wear no other form of pant and (b) there was nothing else at the strip mall that they were interested in. My phone buzzed. It was Dr. Kent.

"Just calling to check in on your postsurgery and see how you're feeling."

"I'm healing up great," I told him, "but my taste is still gone."

"Yes, yes, that can happen."

"How long will it be out for?"

"It can be a few months."

"A FEW MONTHS?!" I damn near collapsed right there on the floor.

"Yes, but give it time. Most people get their taste back."

"*MOST?!* Why didn't you tell me this?" I asked him angrily.

"I definitely spoke to you about it in our pre-op appointment."

I didn't believe him. He sounded like he was just covering his ass. *If I had known this, I don't know that I would have had this operation,* I thought to myself. *MAYBE A CALL TO LAZLO OSWALD IS IN ORDER HERE.*

"I don't remember you telling me this, Doc. All I remember was you telling me about the risk of dying." This was true. That was all I remember, but not all that I had been told. And I had already shown a knack for letting other vital imformation slip through the cracks of my memory. Whatever additional information Dr. Kent had given during our initial consult had blown right by me. And that had nothing to do with my loss of hearing or my brain damage. I had just ignored him. I was too horny for ear surgery to pay attention to anything else he had said.

"I did inform you of this," he said flatly. He then explained, as he had in the recovery room, that the CN7 nerve, which controls taste, goes through the ear on its journey from your tongue to your brain. Mine was now compromised. Turns out all of your senses are physically connected. Who knew?

"In your case, you had a very narrow canal for that cranial nerve, which made it difficult to avoid."

Motherfucker, are you blaming me for my anatomy?

"Is there anything I can do to bring it back faster?" I asked him.

"Just keep tasting."

That wasn't a good enough answer. I emailed the Monell Center to ask if they knew any other, faster remedies. They replied:

Mr. Magary,

It is my understanding that the chorda tympani, which carries taste information from the anterior ⅔ of the tongue, can be injured during cochlear implant surgery. Unfortu-

nately, I don't know of any medical therapy that facilitates recovery from such an injury. Since you presumably had unilateral surgery, taste on the contra lateral side of your tongue should be unaffected, or perhaps even enhanced, but I realize that may not provide a fully satisfying eating experience.

It did not. I was devastated. There was knowledge in my palate I stood to lose. I'm not saying that like I'm some famous chef. This is true of everyone. Within your taste buds are memories, ideas, and the ambition to taste things you've never tasted before. Now I was faced with the daunting prospect of trying to keep all of those taste memories vivid, straining to hold them close to the surface of my mind like they were sunken pool toys. I felt extinct.

We went out for pizza after shopping. The kids were psyched to be eating out for the first time the whole week. We walked into the restaurant and it was too noisy for my ailing ears. Cocktail party effect, etc. The kids loved the pizza. To this day, if Colin sees the phrase "wood-fired" on the storefront of any pizza joint, he wants to go inside and loot the place with his eager mouth. I, in contrast, couldn't taste the pizza at all. I knew what it was *supposed* to taste like. Crisp crust. Tangy sauce. Cheese that's too hot but you want it that way. I didn't get any of that. All I got was a session of dead chewing. The kids ordered ice cream, and it tasted like thickened water to me. I tried to will the flavors into my brain. I had already lost my smell and all the attendant subtleties in taste that came with it. I had lost smoked foods. That had been punishment enough. I was not willing to lose any more of my mind.

But what was done was done. All I could do now was wait and pray that some, if not all, of my senses would come back to me. *This surgery better have been fucking worth it,* I thought. Because as it stood now, without the cochlear implant activated, I had lost over half my face. I was living through cruel game-night hypotheticals. Would you trade an ear for a tongue? Would you trade a nose for an eye? Would you sell your ability to taste ice cream again for $300? I had two eyes, one ear, no nose, and barely any tongue.

I could barely look around the restaurant, I was so dismayed. Everyone else in the joint was eating and laughing. They could taste. They could feel. They could *be*. *They're fine and they have no idea what's going on in my head*. I got up to use the pisser so I wouldn't have to look at the food for a bit, and so that the rest of my family could enjoy their meal without Dad going full goth at one end of the table.

We got back to the house, grabbed Carter, and headed for the beach. I couldn't see the water yet, but the kids could smell it. They quickened their pace as the scent grew stronger. For her part, Sonia would gladly wait all day for twilight to cradle the beach. She's a painter. She majored in art history. In high school, she got accepted into an art scholar program in Colorado Springs that topped her résumé and got her into college. Her paintings adorn every wall of our house in Maryland. One time she painted a portrait of Rudy, and it was like seeing my son ten years into the future. He looked not only older but hardier. Like he had seen so much more than he already had. She had a vision of Rudy in her head that she could only have ever shared with the world via canvas. She saw the contours of his face and the light hitting him in ways that I never could have, despite my seeing the boy every day for over a decade.

That's the gift of being with another person. They see the world—"translate" it, as Sonia put it—differently from you. And when they share that translation, *you* see the world anew. I always thought of the beach at sunset as party time. Sonia knew that the party was beside the point. It was the softening daylight coursing its way through the grassy dunes, the shadows casting every ripple of sand into stark relief, the skimboarders feverishly attacking the surf, getting off a few more rounds before darkness fully envelops the sea. All the world was a painting to her. To see it through her eyes was its own statement gift.

Carter was afraid of the ocean. He remains a strange beast. He still sleeps in a crate because open spaces still intimidate him. He's terrified of other dogs. And he doesn't trust large bodies of water. To this day, we still don't know if Carter can swim or not, and he'll never let us find out. When he saw the entrance to the beach on our evening walk, he pulled back. Dewey Beach allowed dogs after 5:00 P.M. Carter did not view that law as a welcome one. *Oh, no, you can't make me go there.*

"Come on, Yums!" Flora cried. "Come on!"

She gave him a tug and he relented. Carter was like a kid who has to be dragged into something before fully embracing it. The second we got to the end of the path and onto the wide expanse of sand, he blasted off like he was chasing a mechanical rabbit along the rail of a dog track. He didn't know where the fuck he was running, he just knew he wanted to go there FAST. Then he circled back to us and did it all over again. If the waves got too close, he bolted back toward the dunes. The kids never stopped laughing.

We spotted a bonfire in the distance. Volunteers from town were handing out sticks and free jumbo marshmallows to roast over a burning scaffold of firewood. We walked to the bonfire, the kids dipping in and out of the surf along the way. Right in front of the dunes was a line of lifeguard chairs that had been pulled back after the guards had clocked out for the day. Flora, Rudy, and Colin climbed up each one and leaped off. If you have more than one kid, you know that managing the dynamic between your kids is sometimes harder than managing them as individuals. But every so often they stop beating the piss out of one another and become actual friends. Our three kids were being friends right now. I could see it. I still had my two eyes. I saw their joy and their youthful carelessness. I remembered when I could be young and careless. It was a profound luxury, to jump off a chair from six feet up and have no concern at all that anything bad will happen to you. You lose that carelessness as you grow older. Middle age is just a series of physical and mental fires you have to extinguish. But when you steal a glance at young freedom on occasion, you can live inside of it. Your kids are your new youth.

We got to the fire. I couldn't smell it unless I got close enough to lose both eyebrows. I couldn't smell the briny ocean water, either. I toasted myself a marshmallow and couldn't glean anything from it besides the stickiness. But the view of everything around me was enough. I took special vitamins to prevent macular degeneration, because it runs in my family. I needed those eyes. I needed to see. To feel. To watch bonfire embers glowing in the firelight, taking on such deep heat that anything near them would burst into flames on contact. To feel the cooling beach sand between my toes. To see Carter smiling wide after exhausting himself chasing nothing at all. My brain, already forced to do so much remodeling, might have to rewire itself yet again, to smell through sight and taste through touch. I wasn't ready for that yet, but the twilit joy of the beach made the prospect a little more tolerable.

For the rest of that week, my tongue remained semicomatose. The best thing I ate was a side of Rice-A-Roni, which hit every remaining operational taste bud. The wonders of processed sodium. The front of my tongue sensed nothing apart from touch. The back still had some life in it. If I shuffled the food around in my mouth while I was eating, I sometimes hit paydirt. Otherwise, everything tasted disappointing. Cookies tasted like rice cakes.

We got back home to Maryland and I kept on tasting. I had to. Taste dysfunction, as you might have surmised, comes with its own battalion of side effects: side effects that many COVID victims, as with smell loss, would experience firsthand during the pandemic.

Taste dysfunction can make you depressed and insular. Also, if you can't taste anything, you might be prone to eating less, to the point of malnourishment. I went the other way. I figured that if I could only taste 10 percent of my food, I could get the full amount of flavor if I ate ten times more of it. This math turned out to be faulty.

My Deadspin colleague David Roth told me to look on the bright side. "This might be your time to get into mayo," he said. I still avoided it with a fierce hostility. I did try straight buttermilk, though. It tasted nasty, which was oddly encouraging.

I kept noshing, hoping that *this* would be the day my taste came back. When it didn't, my brain filled in the memory of flavor after I'd eaten yet another colorless meal. So I didn't taste the steak while I was studiously consuming it. But then I'd think about that dinner a couple of hours later and the flavors would, to my everlasting wonder, be there. Did that mean the flavors were real? After all, if you listen to Descartes (and don't we all?), the only reality you have is what you perceive. If I adhered to that philosophy, maybe I could live with this sea witch's curse.

But I didn't want to. I wanted to taste a fucking steak again. In real time. If I could have put the brakes on my brain rewiring itself, I would have. But I couldn't. That store never closes. I could still taste sour and bitter things, which is NOT a great combination of flavors when isolated.

On the morning of September 15—I marked the date down when it happened—I was in the kitchen when I grabbed a handful of honey-roasted peanuts. At this point, I was eating things just because they looked good to me, and letting my memory fill in the blanks afterward. I wasn't certain I'd eat a memorable meal ever again. I had spent that week thinking about great meals I'd eaten before flavor had become an apparition. When I was a kid, my folks bailed on a traditional Thanksgiving and took us to Chinatown in New York, where we ate Peking duck with an old family friend who has since died. He ordered everything for us in Cantonese. The food never stopped coming and I never stopped eating. I didn't even know what part of the duck I was eating at certain moments, but that hardly gave me pause. I remembered that duck. I remembered all the pizzas Sonia and I had eaten in New York whenever we had gotten laid off. I remembered the taste of cheap, shitty beer. I remembered lobster. I remembered room temperature lo mein. I remembered the time I smoked a whole Thanksgiving turkey and somehow didn't fuck it up. You truly are what you eat, and after implant surgery I was terrified that my eating life was now at an end and that my tongue would be stone dead forever.

And then I ate those peanuts.

I thought nothing of it for a moment until I was like, *Hey, wait a second. . . . I can taste these.* I got the sweet honey lacquering. I got the salt. I got the peanut grease slicking the back of my tongue. I got *flavors.*

I was up early and no one else was in the kitchen, so I furiously experimented. I ate some dry cereal. Nothing. I ate a spoonful of sugar. Straight, no chaser. I got some of it, toward the back of my tongue. But was I getting it all? I wasn't certain. I sipped a teaspoon of fish sauce and HOLY SHIT, was that salty. I should have diluted that a bit. I opened up a tub of ice cream. Nothing. There were remaining dead patches all over my tongue, but I couldn't ascertain which patches controlled which flavors.

I knew that the front of my tongue was still compromised. My first taste of anything took a beat to register. When you bite into a slice of cherry pie, you get a sugar rush right out of the gate because the front of your tongue gets soaked in all that red-dyed goodness. In my case, I was only getting sweetness toward the back of my tongue, a deep sweetness that needs the sharp sweetness from the driver's seat to help balance everything out. But at least I got a little sugar. Just a kiss.

My adventure with those peanuts was a real-time lesson in what we now know—with a lot of help from researchers at Monell—about how taste works. The old line of thinking is that the tongue has six distinctive, firmly demarcated counties that lord over the primary flavors: salty at the tip, sweet just behind that, umami at the center, two sour patches on either side, and bitter at the back. They used to teach this map of the tongue in schools. In an interview with *Wired* magazine, Dr. Robert Margolskee of Monell explained that the map is a lie, taken from psychological tests conducted by a German scientist and then bastardized into a dopey chart that even children could grasp. Between this and the real story of Thanksgiving, I'm not sure that I was taught a single accurate thing in elementary school.

There is an anatomical cartography to flavor, but it's not necessarily the one you were taught. Margolskee says the front of your tongue is highly sensitive to every flavor, not just the all-pro tandem of salty and sweet. That tip is the bouncer of your digestive system. It can detect, in an instant, if you're eating something that's edible (a Dorito) or something that's poisonous (bleach). It tastes everything, and tastes it perhaps *more* than the rest of your tongue. That's what makes your first bite of pizza so deliriously satisfying. There's no time delay on your trip to Flavortown. You're there the second that pizza hits your tongue and sears it off.

I was still missing that. But I had *something* back. Just as the tip of your tongue can detect the spectrum of flavors, so too can the other parts of it. Whatever I had recovered back there knew these peanuts intimately. They tasted great. It was almost too much flavor, given the epicurean desert I had just wandered across. I felt woozy from all the sensations roaring back into my unsuspecting mind. But if I could get honey-roasted peanuts back, maybe I could still get other things back, too. It had only been a week. Dr. Kent had forecast months of this bullshit. Maybe my high cognitive reserve had other plans. Maybe I could get it all back before my brain rewired itself to accept a life where everything tastes like Styrofoam. I started regularly taking the kids' gummy multivitamins, because I figured any vitamins might speed along the process, and also because they tasted good.

But before I rescued the taste of ice cream and returned it to my now-limited world, I had an appointment to keep. There was something else I needed to get back first.

THE ROBOT EAR

It was time to turn the implant on. I drove to Dr. Morikawa's office myself. No chaperone required. This was not gonna be a miracle, I told myself. Despite missing the hole-in-your-head detail in the background literature, I had read up enough to know that cochlear implants do not instantly bring crystal clear sound back to your brain. Dr. Kent also warned me about it before and after surgery. That was one bit of information I didn't tune out. He told me everyone was gonna sound like Donald Duck at first, which sounded like something that would be amusing for exactly ten seconds.

Medically speaking, I was an ideal candidate for a cochlear implant, because I'd had a functional ear for forty-two years and had only been deaf for a relatively short period of time. There are people, children in particular, who get cochlear implants without ever having heard anything at all. Those people face a much steeper learning curve in being introduced to sound for the first time. There's a human instinct for sound that you can see in touching videos of babies getting their implants turned on for the first time. But those children still have so much ahead of them to comprehend. Also, cochlear implants are a controversial topic among deaf people, the thought being that they could potentially render deaf culture extinct in coming decades. And many in the deaf community are adamant that deafness is NOT a disability, certainly not one that needs to be cured.

I had no such reservations about getting my hearing back. My own cochlear nerve was a seasoned veteran of signal relaying and was eager to get back on the job. But despite the assurances that my surgery had gone flawlessly (besides the nick that ravaged my taste), there was no guarantee that I would get my right ear back entirely. I couldn't keep from being excited, though. *Will I understand words? Music? Will people sound different to me with this new ear? What will their new voices even be?* I couldn't wait to find out the answers, good or bad.

I arrived downtown early. Not wanting to spend more time inside a doctor's waiting room than I already had over the past year, I burned the clock by visiting a nearby Trader Joe's. I grabbed a free coffee sample in a tiny cup better suited to hold ketchup than any sort of beverage. I did my little shot and could taste it. Just the wiring I needed. I went into the Georgetown Department of Audiology and asked if they validated parking. They did not. Insurance should cover your goddamn parking.

Dr. Morikawa escorted me into his office and brought a tote bag (that I could keep!) full of implant swag for me to unbox, all of it gratis. There was the sound processor, called the Rondo. That's the receiver you stick to the side of your head. The microphone inside the Rondo relays sound from the outside world to the implant nestled under your scalp, which then passes it on to an array of electrodes that snake all the way through the cochlea.

This was my new ear.

Dr. Morikawa connected the Rondo to his laptop to program it, matching it to my hearing loss. Same as with a hearing aid. He stuck the processor to my head, parting my hair to make sure it held fast. The Rondo clung to my noggin for a brief second before sliding off. A wire clip prevented it from dropping all the way to the floor. I grabbed the Rondo and put it back on, looking like I had a key fob glued to my skull. It stayed.

But Dr. Morikawa wasn't ready to turn it on just yet. Bit of a cruel tease.

"Your head still has some swelling," he told me. "That's why it's slipping off."

"I'll look normal again eventually, though, right?" I asked.

"Oh yeah. I used a number three magnet for you, but that's not strong enough to stick. Lemme change it out for a number four."

He gave me the number four and told me to be cautious. If the magnet was too strong, it could irritate my skin. Damage it, even. But I didn't care about my skin. I wanted a MONSTER MAGNET: a magnet so powerful it could rip the implant back out of my head. Alas, this slight step up was the maximum amount of polarity the manufacturer offered.

"Are you ready for me to turn the Rondo on?" he asked.

"Hit me."

"This is just a test. You're not gonna *hear* hear anything yet."

"Okay."

He plugged up my left ear (the good one). I whipped out my phone to pass the time. The day they finally resurrect my dead ear and I gotta fuck around on Twitter while Dr. Frankenstein raises the platform up into the lightning storm.

Dr. Morikawa punched a few more keys and suddenly I heard noises. I put my phone down.

This test was strictly about sound perception. We were easing into the miracle. In the beginning, I would hear only whatever Dr. Morikawa's software played for me. I would have to wait for him to disconnect his computer so I could hear *everything* after that. But I could be patient. Shit, I had already spent nine months NOT hearing through my right ear, and getting better at it. What was another twenty minutes?

Dr. Morikawa handed me a laminated loudness scale: Very Soft, Soft, Medium, Loud, Most Comfortable Loudness (this was a misnomer; it really meant most *tolerable* loudness), and then Uncomfortably Loud. My job was to assign a score from the chart to every sound he played. It's amazing how much of modern medicine is still dependent on your being able to accurately describe what you're feeling to a doctor.

"Remember," Dr. Morikawa told me, "louder does not equal clearer." That reminder should be tacked onto the green room wall of every cable news show. He fed the Rondo a series of randomized sounds to see if I could detect them. I felt like I was in the control room during the recording of a new Radiohead album. I heard beeps and buzzes and swells and thrums and pulses and buggy zaps: the first cries of a reborn ear. It was a delightful jabberwocky of noises being funneled back to my ailing brain. I was not emotional while all this was happening. I was focused. Dr. Morikawa and I wanted to make sure the fucking thing *worked*.

There are twelve electrodes in my implant, designed as a group to mimic the human cochlea. Think of them as piano keys: each one programmed to hit a specific note and pitch and, taken together, able to create a coherent world of melody. The electrodes have to align with the "keys" inside the cochlea, so that the notes strike true. According to the tests Dr. Morikawa had conducted while I was under anesthesia, everything was in tune. Now I would hear the results myself.

First though, let me take you inside the cochlea. It's a cinnamon bun–shaped organ inside the ear that's filled with fluid, along with hair cells that detect vibrations and pass those vibrations on to the cochlear nerve, which interprets them as sound. The nerve sends its findings to the brain for final approval. The inner

workings of the cochlea are, like the brain's, still something of a
mystery to the global medical community. This is because the only
way to study the cochlea's innards is by examining one that's been
removed from a dead person. The problem is that, once a person is
dead, their cochlea drains out and ceases to function. So these implants are modern medicine's best attempt to mimic an active cochlea: to reproduce its known abilities and hopefully mimic some
of its unknown abilities in the process. It's a blind guess, but not an
uneducated one.

Dr. Morikawa tested each electrode at varying pitches, like he
was futzing with an equalizer on an old car stereo. The Rondo, like
my hearing aids, was a smart hearing device. It could modulate. It
knew when to amplify external sounds and when to soften them
to keep me comfortable. It kept the volume at room temperature.

I stared a hole through the loudness scale, grading each bleep
and blorp. Some of the sounds fell between medium and loud. Some
sounds were loud, but were they the *most* tolerably loud? Dr. Morikawa played identical pitches consecutively, and I correctly guessed
they were at the same volume. Some cochlear implant patients can't
necessarily discern between sounds, or even volume levels, on activation day. This wasn't a problem for me in testing. Dr. Morikawa
fed me a jet engine–loud buzz that caused me physical pain, and I
was like, *Yep, yep, that's uncomfortably loud.* We were searching for
the uppermost range of volumes my new ear could tolerate, a neces-
sity given my children's ability to shatter a decibel scale.

As we ground through the tests, my volume perceptions grew
sharper. I got more decisive in measuring every quirk and fart I
heard. Every sound had a crisp snap to it. I graded the volume like
an old lady at the deli counter demanding her pastrami be sliced as
thin as possible.

"You're the best reporter I've had for these tests," Doc told me.
Goddamn right I was. He was genuinely excited. This was true of
Dr. Kent as well. When I asked the latter how many times he'd

performed the implant operation, he told me, "A lot, but I wish they'd let me do more." These doctors were evangelists for the technology, not merely because they stood to make money off it but because they had witnessed, firsthand, the results it had produced.

The programming was complete. Dr. Morikawa disconnected the processor from his laptop.

"Are you ready for me to turn it on all the way?" he asked me.

"I am."

He flipped the switch and the right side of my head crackled back to life. We were in a silent office, but of course, no place on earth is truly silent. Every room, even a quiet one, has its own, subtle ambience to it. Let's say you're in a silent office reading this right now. It's not silent. Listen closer. What do you hear? You hear the hum of a computer fan. You hear the air coursing through the ventilation ducts. You hear those goddamn fluorescent light tubes buzzing above you. You hear the far-off machinations of all the HVAC systems and pipes keeping the office physically operational. Even if your office building has soundproof windows, you probably hear the vague din of the outside world penetrating them. If you heard absolute zero, you would notice the vacuum. Something is amiss when nothing at all can be heard.

I could hear this doctor's office. Too much so, in fact. Every sound coming through the Rondo went off like a lit sparkler. I didn't mind. Fireworks were very much appropriate in this moment.

"Can you hear me?" Dr. Morikawa asked. I could. Ah, but I could see his lips moving when he talked, and that gave my brain a head start on understanding everything he had to say. Sight informs sound, and vice versa. Like my friend Kelsey, I had never realized that before. I had never bothered to.

To up the difficulty, Dr. Morikawa covered his mouth with a piece of plain black paper. My job was to repeat the sounds he was making.

"Ahhhh." He sounded like he was using a vocoder.

"Ahhhh," I said back to him.

"Shh."

"Shh."

"Ooooh."

"Ooooh."

"Mary is going to the fair."

"Mary is going to the fair?"

Dr. Morikawa nodded.

"I can meet you on Wednesday."

"I can meet you on . . . Wednesday."

"Is the sound comfortable?" he asked me.

"I think so, yeah. Can I work out with this on?"

"You should. You should always have it on."

"Can I wear a hat with this thing?" I hadn't considered the hat factor.

"Yes, you can wear it over the processor. In fact, you'll want to wear one over it at the beginning to keep it in place." My hat was now going to be a load-bearing hat.

"We're at the really low end of the programming right now," he continued. "As we go along, your brain will adjust and we'll have to bump the levels higher for you." The volumes I was hearing in that moment would not stay that way. Also, they couldn't be too even. Loud things needed to be loud. Soft things needed to be soft. Even them out and the orientation of your hearing loses all depth perception.

"All right," I said.

"But it sounds good?"

"Yeah!"

"We're having a conversation right now. That's amazing." I had never heard a doctor refer to me as "amazing" in any context, ana-tomical or otherwise. I had spent the entire buildup to surgery and activation dreaming of a working ear, but also remaining patho-logically realistic about it. *This could take a year,* I had told myself. I had girded myself for disappointment. But I wasn't disappointed. I could fucking HEAR, well enough that even the doctor was surprised. And doctors never sound enthused about anything.

Dr. Morikawa dropped the mouth cover and started boxing up all of my shit. I got a medical ID card proving I had the implant, lest airport security try to pull me aside to unzip my head and rummage around inside it. Then he gave me my homework: a list of sites and apps with exercises for me to put the robot ear through. I had to train my new ear for at least half an hour every day. And I would. I needed no extra motivation to reach a place where I could again hear the world as it was meant to be heard.

We were finished. It was time for me to go out and live with two ears again.

"How do you feel?" he asked me.

I broke into a mighty smile, wider than the sky.

"I feel great!"

I didn't cry when I told him that, but my voice broke; one of those moments where you're so overcome with relief and joy that your face has a spasm.

We shook hands and I walked out of his office a certified android. The Rondo fell off my head the second I closed the office door. I stuck it back on, then strolled toward the bathroom and let out a burp that, to my new ear, sounded majestic. My own voice, in my head, was too loud. Now I understood, innately, how Sonia felt being around me all the time. I rubbed my fingers next to the Rondo and could hear the friction. No need for my left ear to do the heavy lifting. I went into the john and my tinkle TINKLED. Like I was pissing on a chandelier. A lot of the initial sound I heard came in white. Time would add color to that. For now, I luxuriated in the static.

The robot ear was hungry for any sound it could find: doors opening and feet stepping and faucets running. My cochlear nerve had been waiting to hear again: a clipped power line shooting off sparks, dying to be reconnected. The idea was that, over time, the ear would settle down and become seamlessly integrated with the hearing on my left side. For now, though, the Rondo commandeered the spotlight, and I was excited to see what other magic tricks it had in store. I was excited to start listening.

THE SOUND OF SOUND

I suck at earplugs. Chances are, you also suck at earplugs, you just don't know it. Dr. Morikawa warned me to use one for my good ear (nonrobot division) at loud indoor events, and to use it right.

"Most people don't stick the plugs in deep enough. This essentially renders the earplug useless."

"How far do I stick it in?"

"You want it so that it's barely visible from the outside, to the point where it's hard to pull out."

That freaked me out. What if I jammed an earplug in so deep that I could *never* get it out? This was my only good ear, man. God forbid I stop it up permanently with a wad of dime-store foam. But doctor's orders are doctor's orders, and I had already experienced the fresh hell of being stranded without earplugs at that one bat mitzvah (Kim and Josh, please don't mind me; that was a kickass party you threw). Dr. Morikawa knew more about my ears than I did. I needed to trade my hearing aid for an earplug if I felt like my ear was in danger at any movie, football game, or party. Or rock concert. The last time I had used earplugs, during a Struts concert downtown, I spent roughly ten minutes trying to jam one into my left ear to get it to stick. Eventually I had to ask Sonia to put the thing in for me. Just like losing my virginity all over again.

I survived that first post-hemorrhage rock concert intact, but I needed to get better at earplugs for my implant therapy. I ditched my pride and googled how to properly insert them. You reach over your head and grab the top of your ear with your opposite hand, gently pulling it away from your head. This opens up the ear canal. Then you roll up the plug like a joint and carefully stick it in there. You need to *feel* it slipping down and tickling the inside of the canal, like a Q-tip gone too far. An oddly gratifying feeling. I should not enjoy cramming shit deep into my ears as much as I do.

Before every daily implant training session, I plugged my left ear and then covered it with headphones, hiding away its organic cochlear functions like I was loading up a safe deposit box. My right ear, seeing as how it was no longer my ear anymore, could remain uncovered. There was a way to send audio directly from my phone to the Rondo, but it proved so unworkable that I just gambled with my clumsy plugging technique instead.

I opened up a recommended therapy program called Angel Sound. A disembodied voice said a word—sometimes a real word, sometimes a nonsensical but pronounceable syllable like "fope"— and I had to guess that word from four different choices printed on-screen. One time it gave me "deaf" as a word to identify. Weren't they so clever. Most of the time, I guessed the word right. Other times I was *way* off. The app issued a correction anytime I fucked up, saying my wrong answer out loud, followed by the correct word.

This was a phonics lesson at its core. I hadn't taken phonics lessons since second grade. It was an enjoyable return to basics. More important, whenever I was wrong and the app repeated those words back to me, they *sounded* clearer. For example, at first I heard "big" when the correct answer was "jobe." Huge difference between those two words, right? That's not the case to an infant robot ear. Before answering, I hit the Repeat button several times to make sure I heard the voice as best I could. I swore it sounded like "big." But then the correction came in and, within my new ear, "big" *became* "jobe." The *B* morphed into a *J*. The short *I* slid into a long *O*. The implant was learning to identify these sounds in real time. I was floored.

I got more questions wrong. There are a great many sounds in the English language, after all. Even sounds that I thought were the same were not. For example, one time I got dinged because I guessed that the voice said "sod" and not "sawed." I fumed at the correction. I was like, *YOU EVIL PIECE OF SHIT APP, THOSE WORDS ARE THE SAME.* They're not. Say them out loud. "Sod" comes through your nose down from the roof of your mouth. The upper lip makes corners when you say it, like you're farting out the word. But "sawed" sits down lower, your tongue vibrating to make a deeper sound. There is less distinction between those two words than there is between, like, "cling" and "barf." But it's those small distinctions that give language not only its breadth but also its personality. Accents flow out of these small differences (nothing I just told you about the phonetics of "sod"/"sawed" will apply to you if you're some Boston asshole). If my implant could learn to recognize those differences, then it could hear everything.

But I had work to do. Months and months of it. At the end of my first full day with the Rondo, I was strangely relieved to take it off. The robot ear had done a lot of work, and my brain along with it. I needed a break from the miracle. In many ways, wearing a processor and/or hearing aids is like wearing glasses. If you wear glasses (or contacts), you think nothing of taking them off before bed and flying blind for a moment or two. Corrective hearing equipment has that same dynamic, only you may not think of it that way, because (a) you don't have hearing loss, (b) unlike glasses, hearing aids can be invisible, and (c) vision loss is so common as to be pedestrian, whereas hearing loss comes across as rarer and thus more profound, even though it's neither of those things. Nearly forty million Americans have hearing loss. That's roughly a third of the number of Americans who need corrective lenses. But forty million isn't a meager number, and it isn't just old fogies in that tally.

The post-op swelling went down and the Rondo stuck to my head with increasing vigor, like a lamprey stationed behind my ear. I liked touching the mic and hearing it scratch. I liked putting on a hoodie and hearing the Rondo brush against the inside of the hood. I snapped my fingers and clapped my hands by the good ear and then by the robot ear to make sure the volumes were equal. I rubbed my fingers by the Rondo and fanned air toward it, to see if it was picking up softer motions. I wasn't sure if my left ear was doing the yeoman's work in these moments. I thought to myself, *Is this working? It doesn't sound weird enough.* But then I went back into hearing lessons and knew, for certain, that the implant was working as advertised . . .

Right up until I dropped it into the toilet.

I went to take a leak. I was so used to the Rondo sticking to my head that I had little compunction about hanging around near toilets with it still on. I lifted the toilet seat and then, because God has splendid comic timing, the Rondo fell off my skull and went KERSPLOOSH down into the bowl.

The good news was that this happened before I had started pissing. The bad news was that my ear was now in a toilet. Frantic, I fished the poor Rondo out with my bare hand, wiped it off as best I could, and then dunked it in a bowl of rice, iPhone style. When it had soaked in the ricey goodness long enough, I wiped it down a second time and, because I am not a terribly picky man, stuck the drowned Rondo back onto my head. It worked, but that did little to assuage my fears. Maybe it somehow had piss inside it. How would I know? I wouldn't be able to smell it. I called Dr. Morikawa and fessed up.

"You can bring it in," he told me, laughing. This was not the first time a patient of his had done something foolish with implant equipment. I was in his office the next day, waiting next to a deaf child who was playing with Mega Bloks and had a processor on the left side of her head. I couldn't imagine the struggles that both she and her parents had endured throughout the implant process. And here I was, checking to see if the Rondo I had nearly flushed away fell under warranty. It did, which was good, because its excursion twenty thousand leagues under my toilet had shorted out its guts and made it impossible to program. Dr. Morikawa had a new one programmed and sent to my house.

I settled into the robot ear. The initial echo from the implant—which made everything sound like it was coming from the opposite end of a very long hallway—died down like ripples in a pond. I noticed that when I scratched the mic, I could feel it in my head, just as you feel it in your head when you dig into your actual ear canal. More than that, the scratching now sounded the same as if I were scratching my left ear. Again, your ear is a microphone. It stands to reason that the sound of tapping an ear and tapping a mic would coincide. I was enthralled. Even now, I still scratch my robot ear for kicks. Whatever buyer's remorse I had over getting the surgery vanished. Dr. Kent was a wizard with a scalpel.

Gifted with a urine-free replacement processor, I stepped up to more advanced rehabilitation exercises. The goal was to close the gap between my artificial hearing and my regular hearing. This is the grunt work of living with innovation. Because of my circumstances, I already had a mile-long head start on many of my implant peers. But through the Rondo, with my left ear corked, the world still sounded like it was coming through a transistor radio. Small sounds, like Rudy's flip-flops slapping against his heels as he walked down the street, were noticeably amplified. Other sounds sounded artificial to me. But what does artificial even mean in that context? Natural hearing involves the carrying of electrical impulses, just as my new hearing did.

I needed to train the ear, and my brain, to make the unnatural sound natural. I needed to subject the new ear to a wider range of speech patterns, ambient noises, and even musical instruments. Angel Sound had exercises where I had to identify an instrument from a brief clip. This was *much* harder than identifying words. I confused a piano for a saxophone and a trumpet for a xylophone. I swung wildly and missed a French horn clue, because I have *never* known what a French horn sounds like.

The next week, I moved on to whole passages of text read aloud. On one website, I listened to a sentence blind and had to pick it out from four choices that appeared on the screen after that. I got sentences like "Fried dough and saltfish is a popular breakfast in Guyana" and "A zestful food is the hot cross bun." I would argue with the latter opinion, dead taste buds or no dead taste buds.

For another exercise, I watched a succession of actors read sentences to me. This time, I was quizzed on the content of each reading, not necessarily on what specific words were said. I got to know these actors well. There was an old lady who sounded like your granny reminding you to visit at Easter. There was a brunette who had an easily recognizable Southern twang. Her twang made everything much clearer. Thank you, twang lady. There was a dude with a vaguer accent that destroyed my odds of hearing him clearly. There was also a bald dude who said shit way too fast and low. I didn't care for that guy. Hated him. Every time he showed up, I winced because I knew I would struggle. I yelled at him. I knew I was supposed to challenge myself, but I didn't like doing so. Same as I'd ever been. Dr. Morikawa explained to me that hearing women would be much easier for me going forward, because of the

difference in vocal pitch. Men would be harder for me to understand, which is true in general but even truer in my case.

You could change speakers on this site so that you could get the
actor you wanted every time out. I kept them randomized both for
my sake and for theirs. You could even *rate* these actors on the site.
Can you fucking imagine how insulting that is to the poor actor?
These people are trying to get TV and movie and Broadway audi-
tions, and they get fucking Yelped when they take an interim pay-
check doing therapy reads. I would sue. I would call Lazlo Oswald
and tell him I gots to get mine.

Another site tested the implant with clips of TED talks. Hard
fucking pass. Dr. Morikawa also suggested audiobooks, so I tried
Tom Sawyer to be ambitious, and because I had never read it. I
got bored after a few paragraphs and watched stand-up comedy on
YouTube with the subtitles on instead. I read out loud to myself.
I watched YouTubes of people reading board books for children. I
did exercises on another therapy site—almost certainly designed
for child patients—that featured an animated penguin enthusiasti-
cally clapping anytime I nailed a sound. Those were all far better
alternatives to hearing Doobla CEO Payden Farst lecture an audi-
ence about the future of linear content.

I enlisted the kids in my therapy. I stood across the room from
Colin and had him shout random words to me to see if I could nail
them. Mad Libs without the Mad Libs.

"Poop!"

"Poop."

"Fart!"

"Fart."

"Buttcheek!"

"Okay, I see what you're doing here. You're definitely my son."

I picked him up and gave him a big smooch on the cheek. Colin
gave me a monkey hug, wrapping his arms and legs around me and

squeezing as hard as possible. He was gonna be too heavy to pick up soon, so I had to get my monkey hugs in while I could. Like every other kid, Colin is affectionate but with ulterior motives. He hugs me before asking, with maximum feigned innocence, if I can buy his sorry ass an Apple Watch. Then I say no and he comes back with more love and another request for free shit. But this time, Colin was hugging me just to hug me.

Or so I thought. He giggled and tugged at my hat. Whenever I wear a hat, Colin wants to yank it off. He didn't realize that, this time around, it was securing precious cargo. I yelled like a car was about to hit us.

"Colin, NO!"

He yanked my hat off and the Rondo went flying to the ground. I still had mild PTSD from the toilet incident, so I was prepared for the Rondo to shatter into a zillion pieces like a piece of peanut brittle hitting the ground. But it held up just fine.

"I'm sorry, Dad."

"It's all right, man. You just scared me there for a second."

"Are you still a cyborg?"

"You better believe it."

I settled into life with the implant. My echolocation was back. I could tell where sounds were coming from. I didn't lose my shit at dinner when all the kids talked at the same time. I wasn't as dizzy when I got turned around playing soccer with Rudy. I read to Colin at night with the Rondo on and Carter hanging out in the bed. I could hear my own voice in full. I didn't have to turn the volume way up on movies to grasp the dialogue. I was still too proud to turn on the subtitles on Netflix, which was stupid because that's something a lot of *non*deaf people, Flora included, do (and frankly, as a deaf person, the practice offends me). But now I didn't even have to consider the subtitles option unless I ran headlong into thick Scottish brogues. I could handle crowds without the dreaded cocktail party effect rearing its head. The white noise accompanying everything faded. If I heard an aggressive hair dryer (all of them) going to town in the bathroom, *that* was still overwhelming. But otherwise, I was hearing. The robot ear was its own part-time job, but the training was paying off. I walked outside one night and heard crickets. Real crickets. Not a recorded therapy program. They chirped so loud and so sharp, I started laughing because it felt so good to hear them. Hearing can be meditation, too.

And music came back to me, even after my clumsy attempts to identify the dulcet tones of a French horn. As my PT Ann had foretold, my brain was rewiring itself. The music I had once heard only on the left side of my head was migrating farther inward, closer to the center (in a stroke of "luck," a study conducted on over three thousand newborns concluded that your left ear is better than your right at hearing music, and thus I had been spared my golden ear). The notes were getting clearer. I didn't need multiple spins to grasp a new song. I was inside every song again, and vice versa. This didn't happen overnight. The migration was so gradual I didn't even notice it happening. Now music and I were together again like nothing had happened, which is good, because if I had lost music, I would have felt like I had lost yet another part of my body.

I went back to Dr. Morikawa for a tune-up. The more my brain got used to the implant, the softer the sound coming through it became. This was "normal." Common for members of the implant club. He jacked up the bass and treble. I told him that I could feel something clicking inside my head when I attached the Rondo. It's one thing to have an IT problem, quite another when your wireless router is located under your scalp. Again, Dr. Morikawa told me this was "normal." I was a touch skeptical. If you felt a bunch of shit moving around in there, you would be too.

Dr. Morikawa walked me into the sound booth for testing. Every time I stepped inside, I wanted to lay down vocals for a bluegrass record. Instead, the doctor asked me to identify a series of distant beeps and bloops. He told me the ideal setting for the Rondo was at about 80 percent of the hearing capacity of a normal ear. If he optimized it any further, I would go insane. It may sound like a superpower to hear a squirrel grubbing on an acorn from a hundred yards away, but it's not. It would piss you off.

"I think I know the answer to this already," I told the doctor, "but this will never sound *perfect*, right?"

"It'll never sound perfect." I was ready for that. I had a daydream that the Rondo would come to hear exactly as well as an analog human ear could, but it had already worked far beyond my deliberately tempered expectations. When I had it on, the world felt full again. Sonia told me that my mood was improving. This was the fix that could fix it all.

"Doc, how do you do implants for people who aren't all the way deaf in an ear? Do you have to purposely deafen that ear all the way to make it work?" Imagine having to take *that* gamble.

"There are hybrid implants that work with existing hearing."

"Huh!"

The testing beep volumes were so low that I had to fight my mind to discern if I had heard an actual sound or just a mirage. I didn't fully trust my own hearing, but I tested well. Dr. Morikawa jacked up the volume and asked me to rate the sounds on the loudness scale. He reminded me once more that volume and pitch are not the same thing. Higher-pitched sounds—think of a glass-shattering note held by a soprano—can *seem* louder than their lower-pitched counterparts but aren't necessarily so. Think of the difference between bass and treble. Loud treble splits your face open. Loud bass makes your whole body quiver. Same volume, different effect.

This is the architecture of sound. In the time between my accident and my implant, I took stock of acoustics, because every nuance to them had a pronounced effect on both my emotional and physical states. Now I got to experience those same acoustics from the other side of deafness. I noticed what I could withstand, and I noticed all the astonishing subtleties within sound—entire atmospheres of resonance—as my brain set about rewiring what it had already rewired. It was picking up those subtleties with impressive speed. This is not necessarily common. I have a friend named Kevin who got an implant that straight up did not work. Everything sounded fuzzy and never got better for him. He lost his taste too and never got *any* of that back, either. Once again, I had lucked into the most favorable outcome.

But my luck was hardly blind. I think about all of the circumstances surrounding my hemorrhage, and it's clear that I had an insane number of advantages on my side. I had insurance when it happened, and that insurance actually deigned to cover things. I was surrounded by people who saw me on the ground and furiously rushed to my aid. I collapsed in New York, which has no shortage of capable brain surgeons and was not overrun by coronavirus at the time. I had a family. I had money to pay my deductibles. I had bosses willing to put my family up in an Airbnb for a whole month while I recovered. I was in the most favorable position possible to have the most favorable outcome. What if I had collapsed alone? In fucking Nebraska? What if Megan Greenwell hadn't been at the hospital with me all that night, begging doctors to give me a second look? What if I had *not* had insurance? I know damn well I'm an exception to the rule. I know damn well that, in the grand scheme of the American system, my survival was a luxurious anomaly.

And so was my robot ear. It was almost—and this is a very large almost—as if I had never lost my hearing at all. Sometimes when I'm sick with a stomach bug, I worry I'll never get better. Then I *do* get better and instantly forget the depths of that despair. It's as if I had never been sick at all. Sometimes I forgot the Rondo was on my head, except when I had to piss. I was working through a new and strange phase of amnesia. But this time, I didn't need to bash my head in to experience it.

AMNESIA

I was chasing the ghosts of feelings. In terms of sound, I had managed to recover more than I had ever thought possible. My smell, however, was still on life support. I couldn't bring myself to do smell therapy any longer. I know that comes off as both insane and lazy. We're talking minutes out of the day to potentially recover a critical sense for the rest of my life. But I wasn't getting anything back. The fact that it could take years for my smell to return didn't make me more determined. It left me drained. Every time I took a whiff of clove and got nothing, I felt like the entire exercise was worthless and stupid.

Because it probably was. All that time I had spent sniffing at nothing was depriving me of the chance to rewire my attitude and live comfortably as a scentless apprentice. I could've kept up the therapy and reminded myself that there were no guarantees. But how much (unpaid) work would you want to put into a task you knew would likely prove futile? Would you keep putting together a piece of IKEA furniture if half the parts were missing and they didn't offer any refunds? Fuck and no, you wouldn't. I can barely be bothered to do that shit when I have *all* the parts at my disposal.

There is a very specific cruelty in knowing that, from a medical standpoint, you have to relentlessly keep after your damaged senses if you want to preserve your chance to restore them, while simultaneously knowing that such a pursuit actively prevents you from accepting what could be inevitable. I had to take stock of my nose's long-term odds and decide if I was investing my time—which was now limited in pronounced ways—effectively, or if I was Sniffaphus, cursed to roll a giant jar of eucalyptus oil up a mountain only to have it crush me over and over again.

I began losing smells for good. Again, there was no way to jog my olfactory system by smelling things. Deprived of that ability, the memories faded like an old Polaroid photo left out in the sun. I can barely remember what poop smells like. I know it smells bad, obviously, but the distinct facets of its badness are drifting out of my cortex. I can't even describe those facets to you in writing anymore, particularly given that fecal matter has its own range of smells. If my nose came back, so would every last memory of everything it ever encountered, and then I would forget what it was like to not smell anything. But as it stood, those memories were sinking beneath the horizon. My brain wasn't strong enough to keep them anchored in its harbor. I was surrendering, and disappointed in myself for doing so.

Taste was another matter. Food is a large part of your identity, and I wasn't ready to let that die. My taste was my personal history. It spanned from my being a lonely, overweight child in Minnesota, nuking Lender's bagels and topping them with cream cheese, to my being a full-grown adult and biting into a Korean taco for the first time. I'm the sort of person who builds his entire day around eating—especially without alcohol on hand. Half of all conversations between Sonia and me involved dinner planning, and neither of us minded it all that much.

Our marriage had its own vast culinary history. There was chicken paprika, the first dinner Sonia ever made for me. There was the night she tried to make her own gnocchi, failed, and then swore to never make it herself again (and never did). We called it the Gnocchi Incident. There was the time she introduced me to blue-crab feasts in Maryland, where you smash open a bushel of steamed crabs and pick apart their insides. There were random road stops at Denny's with the kids. God, they loved Denny's. Any place that serves its fries quickly, man. Our life together was a long and impossibly sumptuous buffet.

One morning late in September, I made popovers for breakfast. It's an easy recipe, as far as baking goes. You mix together some flour, eggs, milk, and melted butter, and HEY PRESTO! You got popovers. The kids laid waste to the tin, but I made sure to reserve a few for myself. A standard dad tax on all edible goods in the household. I filled one popover with peach jam and took a bite.

I could taste it. I hadn't tasted fruit in over a month. Suddenly, the bright sweetness of jam was all over the middle and back of my tongue. I ate the rest of my supply in an instant, and then I did another round of Can Dad Taste It?, licking whipped cream off my hand (yes), digging into the ice cream (no), eating a fistful of dry cereal out of the box (no . . . WTF, man), and housing some plain bread and butter (oh my fucking God, yes). As with the miracle peanuts, the returning flavors were almost too strong, because it had been so long since I had experienced them.

I went to the store and bought some fried chicken. This wasn't legendary fried chicken like you'd find at Publix. This was just regular-ass fried chicken. It was the best thing I'd eaten since the hemorrhage. I would remember this fried chicken. Again, I hadn't gotten all of my mouth back, but I had gotten *something*. A taste, if you will. The front of my tongue was still profoundly crippled, but the back and sides were fully out of their slumber. I told Sonia and the kids the good news and they were happy for me, but they could only empathize so much. It's nearly impossible to understand these losses unless you've experienced them yourself. You can't just tell the front of your tongue to shut the fuck up so that you can see what it's like. This struggle was strictly my own. But the small victories I was notching were already proving more than worth the fight. I wanted all my taste back, tip of my tongue included. My nose might have been a lost cause. My mouth was showing that it still had a lot of potential.

This was just in time, because my best friend, Howard, was getting married in October and his bachelor party was in New Orleans. It would be my first time ever visiting the city. I wasn't gonna be able to drink in New Orleans, but I sure as fuck was gonna eat. And see. And hear. I was too old now for standard bachelor-party debauchery. Pretty much all of us were. My dirty thoughts were reserved exclusively for gumbo this time around.

This was my first flight since implant surgery and, to my dismay, the implant didn't set off the alarm at the TSA checkpoint. Before I walked into that glass chamber that does the invisible stop-and-frisk, I told the agents I had metal inside my head.

"That's fine," they said.

"Do you need to see my card for it?"

"Nope."

"Oh."

I landed at the NOLA airport and took a cab deep into town, past all the vast graveyards lining the highway. From an eyewitness perspective, I would never know how close I had gotten to joining all of those angels just ten months prior. I wasn't here. I was someplace else. Unlike everyone who witnessed my demise, I never had the chance to be frightened.

As I recovered, I engaged in a second, more deliberate phase of amnesia. I never looked at my medical charts from the accident. I never looked at the photos my sister took of me in a coma. I never looked at Sonia's CaringBridge entries. This negligence was part of my grand plan to return to my previous self. But also, I was scared. I didn't wanna see how close I had come to death, because I was afraid that once I knew, I would think of nothing else. I would be my own ghost until death came back around once more. There was a dark underbelly to being grateful for living, and for a very long time I hadn't been able to articulate it. If I spent all my time feeling lucky to be alive, I'd really just spend it thinking I *should* have been dead. Because I should have been. Your odds of surviving a subdural hematoma are roughly fifty-fifty: Anton Chigurh flipping your quarter and demanding you call it. And everyone who saw me at the time thought that even *those* odds were inaccurate. The car should have been totaled, man. I feared my fear of death overcoming me entirely.

But then I thought more about my death, and that fear dissipated. I remembered nothing of my coma. I had no out-of-body experience. I didn't have visions of wading along a cosmic seashore next to rainbow-striped dolphins. All I got was black. A power nap. It wasn't anything like the romanticized portrayals of death I'd seen in TV and movies or read about in firsthand accounts of people who had visited the Other Side and lived to tell the tale. There was nothing. *I* was nothing.

I have feared this nothingness for far too long. When I was a child, I asked my parents about death. Mom reassured me that I wouldn't be dying anytime soon. Still, I worried. I *would* die at some point. Everyone and everything would die: mankind, the Earth, the sun, the universe itself. All of it consigned to the void, forever and ever. Worse, I feared I would be *conscious* inside this forever as it stretched on and on.

My whole problem was that I thought about death in terms of measurable time. But this is oblivion we're talking about. My two weeks in a coma went by in the span of a microsecond. And if two weeks could pass by that quickly, how long would a billion years take? I can't be afraid to be dead for a million years when there *are* no years in death. All of the restraints that govern terrestrial existence are gone. There's no time. There's no space. You're not even human anymore when you die. Nothing there exists on a measurable scale. You're something else when you go, and your human form won't be around to piss and moan about the transition. For two weeks, I existed outside of the universe. It was lovely. No paperwork. No scrolling through Twitter to discover new horrors with every flick of my thumb.

If you wanna believe there's a heaven, that's all right. It doesn't matter to me either way. Maybe I saw nothing but black because I hadn't done enough to earn God's mercy. But I suspect that I fell into the black because that was what was always going to be there. I liked it. I don't remember being worried about my coma *while* I was in a coma. I was too gone for that. There's an old Guns N' Roses song called "Coma," featuring lyrics that Axl Rose wrote down after OD'ing four years prior to its recording. His was not a rock star coma. No visions. No pearly gates. Like me, Axl got the express coma, and then he wrote:

I wish you could see this, 'cause there's nothing to see.

Yup. That was my view out there, too. If you fear nothing—if you fear that you will be consigned to an eternal black void—keep in mind that a lot of healthy people meditate on a routine basis SPECIFICALLY to achieve this state of blankness. No thoughts. No distractions. No dishes to wash. There are no angels playing harps on clouds, either, but in my case I was too dead to care either way. I had seen death, but I had also seen nirvana. I had no complaints about it. Death simplifies everything on a scale you and I will never be able to fathom, not even after we die.

Please note that I remain happy I didn't die that night, nor do I intend to die anytime soon. Axl Rose OD'd in a deliberate suicide attempt. Do not emulate his inadvertent path to clarity. You should keep on living until your body can't anymore. Save the best for last. If you're concerned that your hard drive will be erased when you pass through to the beyond—that you'll carry no memories with you, nor ever see your loved ones again—you're still thinking about death in all-too-human terms, no matter how profound you think that angst may be. Also, you're not taking into account the idea that your afterlife may not be something *you* experience, but rather the sum existential impact you've had on the lives you leave behind. Those who love you *are* your afterlife. They are your soul, and you theirs. I went to the funeral of a family member after my hemorrhage, and the kindly pastor read aloud this passage from the book of John:

> *Verily, verily, I say unto you, except a corn of wheat fall into the ground and die, it abideth alone: but if it die, it bringeth forth much fruit.*

I'm not a terribly religious man. You might think my accident would have caused me to be *more* spiritual, given that I was spared. I had become far more open to ideas about God and the lessons of Jesus after Colin nearly died undergoing surgery at nine days old for a malrotation in his intestinal tract. He slept through *his* brush with death, too. Me? I was the one in the waiting room that time around, living in tears. Gripping on to Sonia's hand like it was a cliff edge. Praying. No atheists in foxholes, etc. Colin survived that surgery. Another most favorable outcome.

But after my own brush with the Reaper, I became *less* intrigued by God, or whatever form a higher power takes. I didn't meet God in my coma, and I didn't need to. When you get to know death as intimately as I have, you start to understand that life and death aren't separated by a hard boundary. They bleed into each other, and seeing that osmosis from inside the black makes you understand how death is something that—on a cellular level—redeems everyone.

The pastor's words struck me as ironclad, Jesus or not. They're also true in the literal sense. Atomically speaking, I'll still be here when I die. My body will decay and the atoms composing me will go their separate ways to become soil and air and maybe even vulture food if I'm lucky. We live among the dead every day. Gravestones are only the most visible trace of them. The dead are all around you, in the ground and in the trees and in the sky. They're there not to haunt but to nourish. Mom and Dad had taken me to an art gallery when they visited back in April. One of the exhibits featured walls painted entirely in glossy, pitch-black printer ink. I saw my reflection in the black, but it wasn't ghoulish. My visage merged into the black seamlessly and grew clearer. Sharper. Light emerging from the dark. Black absorbs all colors. It's a hidden rainbow.

Death and life are not in opposition. So when someone tells you to live every day like it's your last, kindly tell them to fuck off. They're wrong. You should live every day like it's your *first*. Live it like it's your last and you'll just run around like the house is on fire. I don't want a bucket list. I don't wanna live like I'm dying. I wanna live like I'm living. And I want there to be more possibilities left when I die, not NONE. Why rush to tick off all of those boxes? You don't get a fucking gold star from God for that. I know now that I am going to spend the rest of my life incomplete. But life was *designed* to be incomplete. It's not a worksheet you fill out. It's an open platform. You do some things, but you also leave behind infinite possibilities for those in your wake. That's the freedom.

Which is why I went to a bachelor party in New Orleans. I didn't go to Mardi Gras (it was September). I didn't go to a crawfish boil (out of season). I didn't go to a titty bar. I left all of that for everyone else. Instead I ate grilled oysters, sampled NOLA bread pudding for the first time and definitely not the last, and took comfort in a more grounded style of nothingness. I waited an hour in line for beignets, which are just fancy-sounding doughnuts. I do not remember everything about that trip, not because I was brain damaged or because I was high but because I was okay with letting time be disposable.

In the French Quarter, a woman told me that I had something in my hair. She thought it was a leaf or something. It was the Rondo. I thanked her and assured her that what was stuck to my head was supposed to be there.

The noise still cornered me. When Howard and I and the rest of the gang went out for the requisite manly bachelor-party dinner, I had to take a couple of sound breaks to rest my ear. I got irritable on various Uber rides. But otherwise, I thought I acquitted myself well for a dead guy. I even, for the first time since my injury, stayed out late enough to completely run down the batteries in both my hearing aid and in the Rondo. I partied hard. No brain damage ensued.

I was getting better at letting sounds go. I had spent months straining, with great physical and mental energy, to hear all I could. The Rondo lessened that burden considerably, but I also realized that I didn't *have* to hear everything. If I missed a handful of social exchanges, or a few details while Howard recounted the time he shit his pants in an elevator, it was okay. I could leave some noise on the table. Again, life is destined to be incomplete. The sooner you accept that, the more you'll enjoy your little parcel of space-time.

In life, as in death, there is comfort in nothing. My whole life, I feared eternal nothingness for primal reasons that are self-evident in all of us. Then again, what am I gonna do when I finish this book? I'm gonna relax. Know why? Because I get to do NOTHING once it's all done, and I'm gonna savor that nothing. Now, too much nothing can wear you out. Ask anyone who was stuck in

COVID quarantine for months on end, myself included. But there is freedom in nothing. Ask any high school student. Or better yet, ask any group of men hanging out at a bachelor party house in the early morning. Those are some incredible nothing hours. I don't remember a thing about them during that New Orleans trip. I let those moments go without a struggle. Forgetting is not a sin.

As with smells, I was forgetting more flavors, but I wasn't putting up as desperate a fight anymore to reclaim them. All tea tasted like tea to me. Frosted Flakes were only subtly sweet, which is not what you want from Frosted Flakes. Pop-Tarts tasted like cardboard. You might think junk food has no nuances when it comes to flavor. You are wrong.

I also couldn't remember the full taste of ice cream. When I told Howard that I had lost ice cream, he reacted like Carter had died. Fair enough. The flavor was still watered down, and I had lost my original point of reference for what it should have been. I had lost the instant, screaming gratification of that first lick. All I got was a wash of cream. Like hearing your favorite song, but only the bass line. It was barely sweet to me, which makes no sense given that ice cream coats the entire tongue, and given that jam had become very sweet to me once more.

But there was no sense in sitting around *waiting* for ice cream to fully return. I had to enjoy what I could do and what I could feel and not bitch about what I could not. I acquired certain *un*tastes: reorienting my appetites toward textures and things that *looked* appealing. Cookies were not what they used to be to me, but they were still good on these new terms. My brain generously accommodated for these shifts. My attitude was slowly coming around on them as well.

That's a transition you have to make when you're sensorially disabled or, I suppose, if you're newly disabled in other ways. "Things can't be the way they used to be" is a lesson you learn in high school, when Dave gets a girlfriend and you realize you can't be best pals anymore. I had either forgotten that lesson or didn't think I had to learn it all over again. But I did. Maybe I wasn't as grown up as I thought I was. You spend all your life grappling with the idea of finality. When you do, you adapt and embrace your limitations fully, and that makes you freer. That's how you get your identity back, even if that identity is altered from the person you once were.

The man I had been died that night in the karaoke bar. Back down here, this was the only man I could be. I was growing more adept at being him. You can defy your mind when you're young and have it pay off. That wasn't the case for me any longer. I had to accept this new mind and learn to live with it.

But I wasn't all the way there just yet. Here's something I *do* remember about New Orleans: I visited Jackson Square, where street artists sell their wares in rows of kiosks outside St. Louis Cathedral. This is a tourist trap, although the tourist traps in New Orleans kick nearly as much ass as the rest of that city does. I got the idea to buy Sonia a painting. I enlisted my friend Robin in the task of helping me find just the right work of art to bring home to the artist herself, at a fairish price. One of the vendors sold paintings framed with debris reclaimed from Hurricane Katrina. Or at least that's what he claimed. Did I believe him? Oh, you fucking better believe I did. Along the bottom row of his pop-up gallery, I spotted a nighttime painting of a streetcar rushing across Canal Street.

"How much is that one?" I asked the guy.

"A hundred and twenty dollars."

"How about a hundred?" I knew I could haggle. He knew that I would try. He wouldn't have quoted me that $120 otherwise.

"I guess I could go that low," he said.

"What do you think, Robin?" I asked.

"Go for it."

I had the vendor wrap up the painting and then spent the flight home praying that my new masterpiece wouldn't get ripped to shreds by the inner jostling of the overhead bin. I already suffer from bin angst anytime I fly, praying I don't get the short straw and have to check my roll-aboard into the black hole that is the airline baggage-handling system. I had gotten my bag and the painting onto this flight successfully, but now I had to make sure some asshole sitting across from me didn't plop a crate of steak knives down on top of it on his way to the bathroom. To ward off that stress, I envisioned successfully delivering the painting to Sonia and having her marvel at it. *OMG, Drew, you got me a gift? While you were at a bachelor party? My hero!* This would be my statement gift.

I got the painting home and gave it to Sonia. She opened it and stared at it, hesitating for a split second before thanking me. I knew what that split second meant.

"You don't like it," I told her.

"No, no. It's very nice. I'm just very picky about art, you know."

"Whatever." I stomped away. When Sonia pointed out that the painting wasn't a painting at all—it was clearly just a print—I outright denied it. We hung the print in the basement, far from visiting eyes. Every time I saw it, I felt both angry at her for disliking it and disgusted with myself for buying a piece of shit. There would be no generous return policy to salvage any of it.

Once again, I deemed everyone around me ungrateful for my efforts. For *me*, in general. There were obvious-in-retrospect epiphanies I had yet to experience. I was walling myself off from them through a combination of arrogance and deliberate ignorance. I still hadn't gone to see a therapist. My temper remained a loose grenade pin. Howard told me, after our trip, that "you weren't quite yourself." Do you know what it's like to have people tell you that you're not you, and not in the "You looked like you had a bad cold" sense? I thought I was doing better. I guess I was wrong. How far away from me was I? *Who* was I to everyone else? Howard was among many people who waited in that hospital for weeks, scared to death that I wouldn't return to myself. His sister Erica stared at my withered body that month and asked, *Who's in there?* Many months later, I still hadn't given her, Howard, Sonia, or anyone else a good answer.

My injury played a role in this unwanted identity crisis— recovery is never a straight trajectory, remember—but so did outright cowardice. I hadn't gone back and examined Amanda's photos or read Sonia's CaringBridge entries. I hadn't *talked* to anyone in my family, in depth, about what happened to them as I lay dying. I had spent so much time trying to forget what I had been through that I had forgotten, and in some cases not even realized, what *they* had been through. The firsthand accounts of my hospital stint that you read in the beginning of this book? I still didn't know many, if any, of those details yet. All this time I had relied mostly on my own perspective—which is to say, a very limited one.

Think about what a selfish act that is, given what the people I loved had done, and endured, to keep me alive. Death I understood now. But life itself? I still wasn't getting it. I was begrudgingly learning to live with the new me, but not everyone else was. For far too long, I assumed that adjustment was their responsibility.

I was wrong. I had the ability to listen now. It was time I used it.

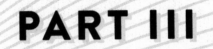

PART III

THERAPY

"**I** HATE THE WORLD! I HATE THE FUCKING WORLD!"

That was me. Alone. In a shopping mall parking lot. I was running a quick errand and short on time. If you've ever been to a shopping mall in the DC burbs, you know that there's never any parking anywhere, and that everyone else driving through the garage sucks. I couldn't find what I was looking for at the mall and then, after sulking back to my car, I got hemmed in by three other cars converging on an open space, leaving no room to get out of each other's way. After waiting—not all that patiently—for the deadlock to clear, I tried to leave the garage, only to encounter one of those surprise dead ends that parking-garage architects put in to keep themselves interested.

I blew up. I grabbed my steering wheel like it was a nurse trying to restrain me and screamed, "I HATE THE FUCKING WORLD!" again and again. When I scream that loud, my voice box jumps out of my throat and becomes a bullhorn.

And I liked it. Anger was a treat I got to indulge in. Anger is seductive that way. I *enjoyed* being angry. Regret came only after the fact. In the moment, there was a little voice in my head feeding me approval, letting me know just how right I was to be pissed.

But this time, raging out in my car, another voice comman-deered my mind. *What are you doing, Drew? What the fuck are you DOING?* I heard myself. I was saying words but they were making no sense. Fury for fury's sake had rendered me unintelligible. I was mortified. Repulsed. I had given myself permission to wallow, and look what it had made me into. After everything Sonia and my family and my friends had done for me—all the crying and all the sleepless nights and all the paperwork and all the begging for me to get up and leave that fucking hospital and live—this was their reward?

This isn't how you repay so much love and bravery. I was a year removed from being a roasted vegetable: a shriveled, blackened, dead thing. Now I could walk again. And see. And feel. And hear. And taste, at a growing clip. I had a duty to these people to be a man worth saving, and I was derelict in that duty. I had forgotten to be grateful for what I had and to love what I loved.

I let out a heavy sigh and drove back home.

All this time, I had balked at therapy. Insurance wouldn't cover it, and I didn't wanna pay full freight. The one thing I clearly needed most, and I was too cheap to get it. I had never gone to a therapist before in my life. This was because I always assumed I didn't need it, which was arrogant. I talked a big game about sup-porting people who spoke openly about their mental-health issues: people who weren't afraid to ask for help. But when it came to myself, I might as well have been stuck in 1950. I figured I was all good. What's more, I assumed that therapy was a racket designed to hook you on scheduling appointments into eternity. You were never "cured," because curing you meant the gravy train would end for your shrink.

But I wasn't all good. When I was in that hospital bed, I told my mom that my brain was the way I wanted it to be. But that wasn't true. My brain still needed help. I was a sour man eager to

pick a fight. I stared daggers at Colin when he came to me with
tech problems. I got angry at speed bumps. When Flora was rude
to me once, I reminded her, "Hey, you know I almost died," like it
was a fair card to play. I yelled at Carter when he barked too loudly
at me. One time I gave his leash a vicious yank when he wouldn't
walk any farther around the block. Cruel people do this. I was
fighting and fighting and fighting, all just to fight, and I was wearing down everyone around me because of it.

"I'm gonna see a therapist," I told Sonia.

"I think that's a good idea." No need to talk this one out. The
second I said I was gonna do it, it was clear to us both that the decision had been long overdue.

I googled around for therapists. I didn't worry about insurance.
I didn't ask for referrals. I didn't look for therapists with an MD
because I had already tried to pill my way out of this, to no avail. I
didn't even restrict myself to therapists who dealt specifically with
TBI patients. I just wanted straight-up, real-deal therapy. I found
a local practice and checked the treatment bullet points on their
website: Anxiety, Depression, Self-Esteem, Anger Management,
Career Changes, Grief and Loss, Relationship Enhancement, and
Parenting. Sold.

I called the practice and they paired me up with Gabriela Bar-
ber, an MS who had an extensive background in treating couples,
middle-school kids, and women suffering from postpartum depression. As an individual patient, I didn't fit into any of those categories. It didn't matter. I scheduled the first available appointment.

Gaby asked me why I needed therapy. I told her that I had
anger issues stemming from a TBI. She explained to me that anger
has five root causes:

1. A need for revenge
2. Feeling helpless

3. Feeling discouraged

4. A need to prove your importance

5. Feeling overwhelmed

Number four. That was me. Every time I got angry at Sonia and the kids, I felt unappreciated and disrespected. *Excuse me, but do I not help out around here? Do I not cook and clean and spend time with the kids and do all of that tedious bullshit without needing to be nagged to do it? You people are lucky I do all that shit. Not every dad does.* That was my internal thought process every time I got mad. I scripted arguing points in my head and then sought out arguments in which to deploy them. I brayed whenever Sonia told me I was overreacting, because I felt like my grievances were not being heard. I wanted to feel *important*.

I wasn't important. I was an asshole.

Gaby asked me if I wanted a name for my condition, just in case filing a claim with my insurance would get me some kind of out-of-network recompense. I did. She marked me down as having adjustment disorder. It was a throwaway diagnosis, used strictly for the sake of bureaucracy. But the phrase stuck in my blotted mind, and a more objective picture of myself emerged. I had a condition. Putting a name to your condition is often its own form of treating it. In my case, I had an affliction from my hemorrhage that roped together every other affliction the accident had produced, a condition that I had refused to notice and hadn't bothered to solve. I couldn't blame Mount Sinai's paper shuffle for this one. This was on me and me alone. I had left my trauma for everyone else to deal with.

Not anymore. I got to work. Same as I did in that rehab ward. Same as I did huffing jars of straight menthol for days on end. Same as I did listening to actors say generic sentences into my cyborg ear. To keep my mind domesticated, I started an Anger Tally in the notes app on my phone, keeping a record of anytime I lost my shit.

For example, one night a smoke alarm went off in the house. The ironclad laws of smoke alarms are that (a) it will always be in the fucking dead of night when one goes off, and (b) you will *never* be able to discern which one is beeping. I hate smoke alarms almost as much as I hate mayonnaise. I couldn't find the culprit. I screamed "FUCK!" so loud and so often that it woke the kids up.

I also included the time I got unreasonably huffy with a CVS clerk, and the time I smacked a wall and hurt my hand because I was in a bus bathroom and the bus wouldn't stop shaking long enough for me to hit the bowl with my piss. They all went into the tally. My own permanent record.

I kept going to sessions with Gaby and grew calmer. More tolerant. More self-aware, in a way that was useful and not just for show. I would not obsess over things that made me feel angry. If I got angry, I would take a twenty-minute "constructive timeout" and distract myself (usually by playing golf on the kids' PS4) so that I wouldn't ruminate on why I was angry about something. In fact, I had to avoid lingering on those issues in *any* way, positive or negative.

Most important, I was learning to get over my own thoughts. Every writer needs to do this and none of them ever do. Not only did I have a writer's ego, but after the hemorrhage, I considered every new thought I had that much more precious. After all, I had nearly lost the ability to think at all. I had to let go of that possessiveness. Talking to Gaby made it clear to me that not all my thoughts were valuable, nor were they useful. I took a clinical look at my thoughts and feelings and then asked myself if those thoughts were helping a situation or not. If they weren't helping, well then I needed to shut the fuck up or seek out helpful thoughts from *other* people. If I couldn't solve the problem after all of that, I had to understand that putting pressure on myself, or on other people, to fix it right away wasn't gonna amount to anything. Some problems—a permanently disabled olfactory system, for instance—have no solution. Your salvation lies in accepting that and adjusting your life accordingly. It does not come from sitting in permanent dread.

"It's okay if we see a path for ourselves but end up on a different path than we were expecting," Gabby told me.

Now, all of this sounds like rudimentary psychology to you. You've probably been screaming SEE A SHRINK since the prologue. But because I had been so stubborn and so ignorant for so long, I had bypassed some obvious truths about mental fitness that could have saved me, and my wife and kids, an incredible amount of angst. Every time I recounted one of my angry outbursts to Gaby, she always knew the *exact* questions I had failed to ask myself during those outbursts. Was I helping anyone but myself while ranting? Was I really listening to other people, or just waiting for them to finish so I could get in my precious rebuttal? I was so embarrassed that these questions didn't come to me in the heat of the moment that I had a hard time confessing that neglect to Gaby. I wanted to lie and tell her that yes, those things had absolutely occurred to me at the time. But I didn't lie. I confessed. And once I did, the neglect ended.

Seeing a therapist was like taking an antidepressant that actually worked. Without thinking about it much, I settled back into myself. Lights were coming back on. Sonia asked me why I felt better, and I couldn't even articulate it. I'm not sure I wanted to look too closely and ruin the magic. I looked back on moments when I was angry and cruel, and they felt so stupid to me. So unnecessary. I didn't need anger to live anymore. I never had.

"Am I getting better?" I asked Sonia.

"Oh my God, yes."

I stopped blowing up at meals. I stopped yelling while in the car. I learned to open my soul to people instead of just *baring* it. There were some things I could keep to myself. And instead of complaining about my own nose when Sonia smelled something, I asked Sonia to describe what was in the air to me—to translate the scent—so I could enjoy the idea of it. If everyone else could smell, why not use them as a resource rather than live in envy of them? I went entire weeks without having to mark something down on the Anger Tally. Weeks would soon become months. I was not cured. I am still not fully cured. I still see Gaby, because I now understand that this isn't a scam. This is routine maintenance for a brain that, while busy getting high on its own high cognitive reserve, desperately needs to stay in shape. Same as my body does. Insurance even ended up covering half of my therapy to boot. Why hadn't I gone sooner? Why why why why why?

I still hadn't looked at the photos my sister had taken of me while laid up at Mount Sinai. She had sent them, with permission, to Sonia—who also never gazed at them—for the sake of record keeping. In case I was ever compelled to look back and see, in full, the damage my own mind had wrought upon me, I asked Sonia to forward me the pictures, which she did from her phone while unloading a few groceries. I walked into my office and gave myself a once-over. My first reaction seeing the photo was *Oh, God, they propped me up. That's bad for my back!* I've had back problems for so long that being mindful of them is always my first reflex, apparently even when there are much bigger problems happening due north of my spine.

I was expecting the photos to scar me, which was why I had avoided them for so long. But where had avoiding things gotten me? I looked hard at the photos. I'm looking hard at them again right now. I'm clad in a dirty hospital gown. I have gauze wrapped around the top of my head. I have a shiner as distinct as Jupiter's Great Red Spot. If you've ever had a black eye, you know that the bruising tends to break away from the eyelid and spread out in unruly directions. But in the photos, I look like I meticulously applied eggplant-hued eyeshadow to a single eye before falling into a coma. I am unconscious, hence no tubes being ripped out. My mouth is hanging wide open. This is my standard dad nap pose, only this time it's an intubation tube keeping my maw pried open. I am un-shaven. As Howard noted, it does my face no favors.

There's a thin, clear tube running out from the back of my head, filled with blood. My nose is plastered with beige elastic tape. There's a single yellow tube—the color of flu snot— running out of it and reconnecting with a tangle of other breathing tubes litter-ing my body. I have so much shit coming out of me, I look like the backside of a TV set.

I was not scarred by seeing these photos. I'm sure it was *very* scarring to see me like this as it was all unfolding, with my life hanging by a wire. But when I opened up the files, my fate was no longer uncertain. Sonia and the rest of my family had to live with these injuries as they were happening in real time. I got to miss all that. Instead, I got to wait a year, open up a .jpg to say, *Oh, so that happened,* and then go have a can of seltzer. I needed to understand what a luxury that was, and I did.

I know people who have had serious heart problems. They've had to live through the terror of diagnosis, surgery, prognosis, and recovery all in real time. Hence, they've come out of the experience with a new appreciation of life. All that carpe diem shit. But I had been unconscious for the first two steps of that process and awake only for the recovery part of my accident. Recovery is slow, painful, and annoying. I know this because I wouldn't stop telling people it was. But I didn't have any *terror* to counterbalance that irritation. I bequeathed that terror to my loved ones, and I remain, to this day, both guilty and heartbroken over it. Selfishly, I remain glad I didn't live through the fear. Anyone would avoid such things if they could. But in my case, terror was necessary in its own way, to temper the frustration I felt with recovery, and with life in general. There was no way to replicate that terror, short of sawing my own leg off without anesthesia or something.

But there was a way to see that terror: Sonia's CaringBridge journal. Now that I had seen photos of myself near death, it was time I read about the ordeal through her eyes. Through her memory. I asked Sonia for her CaringBridge login. All of the entries were spare, like this one:

> *We didn't stay long as they were exhausted from the trip and in various stages of colds. It was hard to see him like that so we all had a good cry at the apt*

And then another, from ten days later:

> *So grateful for our vast network of friends and family who are supporting us with meals, Starbucks, cards, crafts, lunches and all over concern. First day I really know it will all be ok.* ❤

All of the entries contained hints of terror. But it wasn't the terror that stood out. It was the bravery. Sonia went far past the standard human parameters for what even defines it. I saw bravery in every painful step forward she took. Bravery even when no reasonable person would have demanded bravery on my wife's part. Sonia was brave from wire to wire. I read all of her journal entries and realized that I would never, in my life, have that kind of courage. The least I could do to repay that bravery—the absolute fucking least—was to muster some of my own courage and face down the broken man inside of me.

Throughout my recovery, I had failed to do that. Instead, I kept telling Sonia, and myself, reassuring lies. Once I got to X milestone, we would live happily ever after. *Once I can work again* became *once I can smell again* became *once I get my hearing aids* became *once I get implant surgery* became *once I can taste ice cream again*. I always needed something to look forward to. The future was my heroin, because my past and present were not things I was willing to accept. I languished inside needless, obstructive thoughts rather than put in the effort to be the best version of the new me I could possibly be.

Thanks to therapy, I finally began that effort. I saw that it was time for me to accept my new existence. Embrace it, even. I still have no firm answer as to how I nearly died that night, and the mystery of it didn't torture me so much as it left me feeling as if all of this had been so *unnecessary*: a reality I didn't deserve to be living in. A reality I could ignore if I so chose. It's possible, if you believe Chris Thompson's and Bobby Silverman's accounts (which I do), that I could have suffered my hemorrhage *before* falling, and not the other way around. There are four common risk factors for suffering a spontaneous brain bleed: old age, being male, high blood pressure, and excessive alcohol intake. I ticked off at least one of those boxes (being male) when I got hurt, and even though I wasn't drinking a lot that particular night, my lifetime of heavy drinking prior to then almost certainly ticked off a second one.

Even without those risk factors, anyone can suffer a sudden brain hemorrhage, myself included. It's possible that I already had an aneurysm lurking underneath my skull. I've been using the word "aneurysm" wrong my whole life. Anytime I said, "I'm gonna have an aneurysm!" because those clowns in Congress were at it again, I was implying that my brain was exploding. Now that my brain *has* exploded, I can tell you that an aneurysm is not the explosion but rather its prelude. An aneurysm is a bulging blood vessel. The wall of the vessel is distended—either from birth or during the course of life events—and stretched unnaturally thin, leaving it vulnerable and apt to burst at any given moment. An aneurysm is a lit fuse. Perhaps my any given moment was December 5, 2018. Or perhaps someone kicked my ass in a tidy ten seconds or less. Dr. Caridi said he believes "something happened" that night. Even in death, I may never know what that exact something was.

Turns out it was all the *other* shit I didn't know that mattered more.

Because no matter how it happened, the damage was the damage. Now I was looking at its aftermath with fresh eyes and a mind that was aching to heal. I wasn't afraid looking at the photos or reading the journal entries. I was okay. Obscenely so. Not only had my doctors and my family and my friends saved my life, they had saved *all* of it. On my computer screen, I was seeing where I had been. But really, at that moment, I was seeing where I was now. At home. Standing up. Aware. Alive. So many things could have gone wrong. If I had told Bobby Silverman I *did* want a cab ride home that night, I would probably be a dead man right now. Same thing if Megan Greenwell hadn't come with me to that hospital. I was gleaning a deeper understanding of how lucky I had been to survive.

More important, I was finally starting to appreciate how lucky *my loved ones* felt that I had lived. You would have thought that would be easy for me to ascertain after coming out of a coma and being nursed back to health by a heroically patient Sonia. It was not. I had been too damaged and too selfish to understand *why* she put in all that work. That work was love. Every single minute of it. Not only did my wife love me, but she felt fortunate to have me, and I had never considered myself worthy of someone feeling that way. All the way back to my days as a lonely first grader, I felt so, so lucky if anyone *liked* me, much less loved me. The idea that someone else could feel similarly about me was unfathomable. It would have felt egotistical to even entertain the notion. And while my ego certainly grew over time, that parallel insecurity did not fade. I hoped the people I loved loved me back, and I felt overwhelmingly lucky when they did. It never really occurred to me that the feeling would be mutual.

This is true for you too, by the way. The people you love who love you back? They feel lucky to have you. You should know that. I know I do.

NEW YORK

I had a vision of my triumphant return to New York after leaving it in pieces the year before. I would show up at the 2019 Deadspin Awards (but not host them; Sonia asked that I relinquish the mic for that ceremony, and I happily complied). I would see all my old Deadspin friends again. In an act of ultimate defiance, I would even go to the karaoke bar and finish what I'd started. I would sing and dance and show Death that I had emerged from our tango not only stronger but also on key.

But there wasn't gonna be a Deadspin Awards ceremony in 2019. That's because, right around Halloween, I and everyone else working at the site quit after management fired Barry Petchesky—as if the poor man hadn't suffered enough from me vomiting all over him—and demanded that we write only about things they deemed appropriate for us to write about. Also, the CEO was a belligerent prick who had already driven Megan Greenwell to quit for a job at *Wired* in August. Megan's boss, Susie Banikarim, had been laid off even before that. Our site and our careers were being dismantled bit by bit.

On October 30, we hopped on a conference call as a staff, without management present, to talk about Barry's firing. Over the

course of that call, it became clear that it would be the last meeting
we would ever have working together.

"I knew it would end someday," I said to everyone. "I just didn't
expect it to be this way. I don't know what I'm going to do, but . . ."
I couldn't finish the sentence. The tears got to me before the words
did. I handed in my resignation the following morning.

We resigned in spontaneous clusters. Dominoes falling without needing to be pushed. I was in the second cluster. My general
rule of thumb is to never quit a job without having another one
lined up. Plus my family needed health insurance. *I* needed health
insurance. You don't wanna find yourself in an insurance desert
when you have documented brain damage, much less any other
permanent condition. But I quit anyway. I had already started to
figure out life after my own death. I would figure out life after my
job somehow. Deadspin went dark after our exodus. G/O Media,
which now owned the site, eventually hired a new editor in chief
and relaunched the site in March 2020, but no one read it. The site
clearly wasn't itself anymore. As I write this, Deadspin remains
alive but incapacitated. A vegetable.

So Sonia and I made the pilgrimage back to New York for
Deadspin's unofficial send-off: December 12, just over a year after
my injury. No one from the site had seen me, in person, since I
had left the hospital. I do believe we had some partying to make
up for. All of us had resigned, but we weren't about to kill off the
very thing we loved without getting together and drinking (or, in
my case, smoking) the night away. It was time for a funeral of a
different sort, and time for me to reconnect with people who had
last seen me in a hospital bed, unsure if I'd ever get up from it.

Sonia and I came up on the very same bus that she had ridden
up to Manhattan and back multiple times while I was laid up at
Mount Sinai. I had never ridden it before, and now I was kicking
myself for never taking advantage. It was cheaper than a train or a

flight. The seats were nice, the Wi-Fi was shockingly reliable, and the windows were *enormous*. I had never seen Manhattan so clearly. It was a flawless day, and we hadn't even arrived outside Madison Square Garden yet.

We had been young in this city once. We fell in love here. Sonia lived on the fifth floor of a fifth-floor walk-up, above a shitty bar that belched out the smell of wing grease all hours of the night. She hated that smell. But I, a lifelong wing fan, never complained about it. I also rarely complained about the walk up to Sonia's place, because I knew who was waiting for me behind that door. . . . If the walk up had been twenty stories, I still would have happily put one foot in front of the other to get to her. Sonia was where I belonged.

We moved in together in New York, merging our respective circles of friends, drinking pitchers of beer at shitty bars, getting laid off from one cubicle drone job after another, browsing our way through fancy grocery stores on weekends and never buying anything because we didn't have the cash. She bought me a watch. I bought her a ring. She believed in me even when no one else had any good reason to. I trusted her from the night we met, and I never stopped. New York was where we began, where our separate footsteps merged together into eternal lockstep.

The bus came out of the Lincoln Tunnel. Now we would walk the city's streets together again, alive and unencumbered.

After checking into the hotel, I wanted to get some soup dumplings. Then I wanted to go to a shitty Islanders bar in Union Square called Offside Tavern. The Deadspin staff loved that bar's cheesy bread, so I was gonna order a shitload of that and take it with me to the party. Also, I was gonna visit the karaoke lounge, which was still open at the time. Just me. Sonia gave me her blessing but didn't want to step foot inside.

We checked into the hotel and then met Byrd Leavell at a Chinese restaurant for a late lunch. I had not seen Byrd since that car ride back home to Maryland. He walked through the door, clad in his usual tweed suit and vest, and gave me a firm bro hug.

"You look fucking GREAT!" he told me. I didn't object. One thing about surviving death is that you feel beautiful all the time. The standards are lowered. If you can walk and talk and look presentable, you're gorgeous. I was gorgeous. Felt nice.

Then I ate my weight in dim sum and became a touch less gorgeous. Whatever appetite problems I'd had while recovering at Mount Sinai had not lingered. Whatever taste and smell losses I still suffered from were no longer of any concern to me. I still loved to fucking eat. I loved poring over the menu. I loved seeing the food arrive at the table in waves. I loved marveling at the bounty before us now: plates of all shapes and colors, topped with dishes I knew would be perfect before I had even touched them. I loaded my plate with dumplings and noodles, then stuffed all of it into my face, feeling it mix around on my tongue. I still loved the *mechanics* of chewing all that food down and swallowing it. Swallowing is its own pleasure, dick jokes aside. There's a reason you can't chew food and then spit it out to avoid the calories. You have to complete the process of eating by gulping that food down. Then, and only then, does your brain feel satisfied. I had not lost that bit of cognition. No, I hadn't.

We ate so much, and spent so much quality time with Byrd, that time compressed. We had no time to get the cheesy bread. Shit. I wasn't gonna be able to visit the karaoke bar, either. We had to get to Deadspin's funeral in time. In fact, everyone who quit needed to get there an hour early, before all the other guests arrived. We were having a meeting.

The now-defunct Berg'n was a beer hall in Brooklyn that emblemized the pre-COVID dining culture perfectly by doubling as a self-contained street fair with mean acoustics. There were community tables arranged in the center of the space, surrounded by stands operated by separate vendors selling tacos, barbecue, bing

bread crepes, burgers, and, of course, beer. A shitload of beer. I
didn't drink anymore but I did have my weed on me. I could still
party.

Once we arrived at Berg'n, Megan Greenwell took us into a
private room off the main space and told us that, after quitting,
we had received an offer from a holding company to start our own
website. They would give us a generous amount of seed money but
we, as employees, would own 70 percent of the company. We could
not tell anyone else arriving later that night about the offer, nor
did we (many of them found out anyway). Months later, we would
formally name the site Defector, and then launch it in September
2020. We were so hellbent on working together again that when
the promised funding took longer to arrive than we wanted due
to the pandemic, we launched the goddamn thing ourselves. By
the end of 2020, Defector had already earned the same amount of
money that the holding company had initially offered to fund us.

So what was intended to be a funeral was instead a clandestine
baby shower for our new venture. I grabbed Sonia a beer and then
we worked the room. There were Megan and her husband, Dr.
David Heller. There was Jorge Corona, the only person who had
seen me fall but hadn't really seen me fall at all. There was Kiran
Chitanvis, who was quick on the draw with the 9-1-1 call that
spared me from an early grave. After that call, Kiran refused go to
karaoke clubs ever again. She couldn't even walk past them.

There was Victor Jeffreys, who rode with me in that ambulance,
fearing for my life as if it were his own. There was my half-deaf
compatriot Kelsey McKinney, whom I was finally meeting in person for the first time. There was David Roth, who came to the
hospital after my coma with two bags of cold cuts for me. Roth was
embarrassed he hadn't brought any other sandwich accoutrements
with him, failing to realize that eating lunch meat straight from
the bag was, and is, my lifelong passion. There was Samer Kalaf,

who took me aside for a moment during the party and told me how happy he was to see me alive. I'd heard that from Sonia and my folks many times over the course of the year, to the point where I had tuned it out. Hearing it from Samer was an effective reminder. *Oh, right, I'm still alive! Holy shit, how'd* that *happen?*

Everyone was there. I wanted to carve a roast beast, Grinchstyle, and dish it out to all of them. Berg'n lacked that particular stand, alas. I still wasn't certain that I could have a good time without being constantly attuned to my sensory and emotional deficiencies. But being around everyone again was enough to pull me out of my head. I took a couple of sound breaks from the growing celebration, but otherwise I blended into the crowd with relative ease. At one point, I was talking with old colleague Diana Moskovitz, who was unconsciously drifting to my right as we spoke. I adjusted so that my better ear was facing Diana, but she kept drifting. It was like two fifth graders dancing. I was more amused than annoyed by it. I never bothered to demand she hold still.

As in New Orleans, I let some sounds go. If I didn't pick up everything someone said . . . well now, I had been to enough loud bars before I got hurt to know noise in that environment is not a problem solely restricted to the deaf. I forgave myself for not making out every single word coming at me. Besides, everyone else was drinking anyway (and I was stoned). Get drunk at a bar and the words are set adrift. If you can't hear each other through the whiskey and the jukebox, it doesn't really matter. You're loud and incoherent, and THAT is partying hard, my friends.

No good party is complete without an after-party, and my former (and future!) colleagues had the bright idea to hit up a karaoke bar once we were finished at Berg'n. Attendance optional, of course. Both my ears—human and cyborg—pricked up. They weren't going to *the* karaoke bar, but they were going to *a* karaoke bar. I wasn't gonna be able to revisit the scene of my accident, but here was an indirect chance to bring this strange odyssey full circle. To choose my own destiny. Also, it would make a tidy ending for this tome now, wouldn't it? Barging into some unsuspecting karaoke bar, queueing up "You Got Lucky," and singing it until I burst into tears. That would have wrapped everything up nicely.

There was one problem, though: I was exhausted. Sonia was, too. We had been out until midnight already, well past our usual bedtimes. No deafness or brain damage necessary for fatigue to set in. I wanted a nice ending for myself, but it's okay if some stories go unfinished.

Sonia and I bade everyone good night and hopped on the subway. The train stopped at the World Trade Center. The conductor announced the train was being put out of commission, and summarily kicked us off. We had to take a cab the rest of the way. Took over an hour door to door. When we got back to the hotel and got in bed, I never wanted to wake up.

But I did. I had more living to do. I had come back to New York and started over with my best friends, but now it was time to keep things in the family.

CHRISTMAS

2019

I needed a statement gift. This was gonna be my first Christmas out of the hospital since my accident, and I needed to get Sonia something expensive to fit the occasion. Seeing as how I was formally unemployed at the time, we didn't have room in the budget for a "big fucking piece of jewelry," which she had rightfully earned. And I wasn't gonna fuck up and get her a counterfeit New Orleans painting again. So what could I get that was big but also made sense?

Well, Sonia always said she needed a nice handbag, with "nice" being shorthand for "not from Marshalls." I could buy her a handbag. But could I buy her the *right* handbag? You'd never know it judging from who she married, but Sonia is a highly selective person. You already saw how hard it was to get her a fucking watch. Now I was venturing into even fussier territory. I needed help.

Flora. I needed Flora, now thirteen, to be my personal stylist yet again.

"Hey," I said to her, "I gotta talk to you."

"About what?"

"Not here." Sonia was also in the kitchen. When I need to talk to another member of my family privately, without anyone else overhearing, I am NOT subtle about it. Flora and I walked to the living room.

"Can you help me pick out a bag for Mom for Christmas?"

"OHMYGOD YES." Mention shopping or Timothée Chalamet to my daughter and her eyes double in size.

"All right. Let's ride."

We drove to the mall and walked into the accessory section of a fancy department store. They had all the primo shit on display: Vuitton, Coach, Prada. Beverly Hills in an alcove.

"Can I help you?" a sales rep asked us.

"Yes, ma'am. We're looking for a nice handbag for my wife."

"Okay. Did you have a budget in mind?" I gave her a number. She twitched and said, "Well, we have very nice wallets . . ."

We left.

A few days later, I went to the watch repair shop to see the clockmaker and his parrot. I asked him to replace the battery in the Swiss Army watch that Sonia had given me. He said it would be twenty bucks. *That* was within my budget. I stood around awkwardly as he donned his jeweler's eyepiece and set to work. His parrot, with its candy-corn beak, looked away in profound indifference. Five minutes later, the watchmaker handed the timepiece back to me, and I put it on my wrist for the first time in over a year. Looked good on me. Made me look like I deserved to be Sonia's The One.

I went back to the mall, alone this time around because Flora was in school. I walked into a stand-alone designer store and perused the bags. It needed to be the right size. Back when the kids were small, Sonia bought a bag that could accommodate diapers, wipes, bottles, burp cloths, travel containers of baby formula powder, bandages, Neosporin, the Jaws of Life, and an arsenal of other god-awful shit required for even the quickest of jaunts. But our kids were bigger now, which meant that her purse only needed to hold her wallet, her keys, lip gloss, eyeliner, two different tubes of moisturizer, breath mints, sunscreen, and a baby panda. So it had to be big, but not *too* big. It had to be light, but it also needed to be practical and not just some glorified change purse you see women tote around at a wedding reception. I was on a unicorn hunt. It was going to take all of my cognitive functions to trap it.

I gazed at the bags on display. I was forty-three, but I still enjoyed going to the mall to look at crap. Especially *nice* crap. Made me feel like a movie star. I felt along the outside of a sexy red bag and deemed it too garish for Sonia's taste. I groped another bag that was more elegant, but its main compartment was divided by a long zipper pouch. Shoddy interior purse design. It looked fetching, though. And it fit the budget. As a dad, I'm quite adept at reorienting my priorities, and the priorities of others, based on budgetary needs. You already saw where that got me in terms of mental health.

This bag might be worth a shot. And then you'd be done with it.

No. No, man, you've been in exactly two fucking stores so far. Keep at it.

Toward the back, sitting on a lower display shelf, I spotted a finer candidate. Nice, open main compartment. Supple, dark-red leather on the outside. Flashes of snakeskin here and there. Again, within my budget. I gave the salesman Sonia's full consumer profile, like I was sketching her out on paper.

"You think this one works for her?" I asked him.

"Well, what do *you* think? You're the one married to her." Good point.

"I think it works, but I've never made this kind of purchase for her before. I'm not confident, you know?"

"Do you like holding it?"

I slung the bag over my shoulder. "Yeah."

"I might have one that works a little better, but it's expensive."

"How expensive?"

"Eight hundred dollars."

"That's fucking expensive."

"Well, look, I'll knock forty dollars off that one you're hold-ing. And we have a ninety-day return policy. If she hates it, you bring it back and she finds what she likes. But it's not like you half-assed it."

SOLD. I bought the handbag, checking the label to make sure I hadn't bought another knockoff item by accident. The box this purse came it was arguably nicer than the purse itself. I brought the box home and tucked it into the recesses of the laundry room, then told Sonia to not go exploring those recesses. She acceded. Later on, I snuck Flora down and opened the box so that she could gawk at the swag nesting within. There went her eyes, doubling again.

"Look good?"

"I love it."

"Remember, this is for Mom, not for you."

"I want it."

"You're very funny."

There the gift stayed for the ensuing week, unmolested by the Magary women. It was the last thing I packed into the car for the ride to my parents' house. Sonia looked in the back of the minivan, saw the brand label emblazoned across the shopping bag, and let out an *OOOOOH*. I was halfway to success.

We drove over the river and through the woods to my folks'. My parents have lived in the northwest corner of Connecticut for thirty years now. Driving to their house always takes an hour lon-ger than I'd like it to, mostly because traffic near them is inexplica-bly horrific. Then again, it took *them* five-plus hours through traffic to reach me the morning of my brain surgery, so what was my own dread of traffic worth at the moment? NOTHING. I was a good boy for the drive. For the final leg, we cruised along a rural high-way built next to dynamited hillsides that were now glazed in ice. Sleigh bells jingled in my head. I broke eighty and Sonia reminded me to not kill us all. Fair enough. The precious handbag would've gotten scratched in a crash. I couldn't have that.

From their kitchen, Mom and Dad saw our van coming up the steep gravel driveway. As they always do, they walked out the door to greet us as we parked. They had visited our house in Maryland a handful of times since my injury, and every time they came, they looked astonished to see me. It was no different this time. I could see it in their faces: surprise and profound happiness that I was still alive. Out of a bed. Talking coherently. Asking what was for dinner and when I would get to eat it. Mom gave me a fat hug, followed by my old man. Their hugs now last a beat past formality.

On Christmas Eve morning, we took the kids snow tubing at a nearby mountain. It was all of us: Amanda and her kids, Alex and his kids, Sonia and ours. I promised Sonia I would wear a hel-met. The tubing area was off to the side of the main ski area. You grabbed a tube and then stood on a wide conveyor belt: a moving walkway up into a great white expanse. Then you walked to an empty tubing lane, parked your ass inside the doughnut, and flew down.

I set my tube down between Rudy and Colin.

"You boys ready?"

They were already halfway down before I even got a chance to push them. I sat in my tube and shit got real fast real quick. The sensory difference between seeing someone else go fast down a mountain—as I had watched other tubers do during our ascent—and *being* the one who's going fast is hilariously vast. My tube hit terminal velocity and for a split second, I was like, *I better not fall off this fucking thing.*

I didn't. It was an inner tube. Pretty foolproof design.

Sonia watched from the bottom of the mountain. When we

first started dating, I took Sonia to this same mountain to ski with her. I'll never forget her screams. From the top of the slope all the way down, her mouth never closed. She was screaming, but also smiling as a defense mechanism. It wasn't like a kid screaming on a roller coaster, where they're terrified but exhilarated. It was more *Well, I'm gonna die, and isn't it funny everyone will get to watch?* She went down the bunny slope a grand total of one time, her ski tips kissing the whole way down. She never went skiing again.

That was her loss, because skiing and tubing are AWESOME. We did run after run, the kids shedding new layers of gear on each successive pass. I walked over to Rudy and blew sharply down his shirt to keep him from overheating. We were getting some Colorado sun that day. A Christmas gift in advance.

With Sonia's blessing, I did my final few runs without a helmet. My head survived.

We drove back to the house and got ready for church. My parents were not religious, but Mom always made an exception for Christmas Eve. When we were kids, she and Dad dressed us up and then dragged us to a nondenominational service prior to dinner every twenty-fourth. At those services, I fiercely eye-banged the program, ticking off its items one by one as they passed. I stood and sang the carols I knew, snickering with Alex whenever the hymnal forced us to cram two syllables into a single note—one of the off-brand verses of "O Little Town of Bethlehem" is guilty of this—and then I checked out hot girls in the nearby pews. Christmas Eve dinner and Christmas morning were our reward for enduring that barely-an-hour stretch of forced spiritual contemplation.

I, inevitably, grew to love the tradition. I told the kids we were going to church with Gammy this night, and that they would have to dress nice. Every pout they let out was one I knew intimately.

Sonia and I got Rudy and Colin into jeans and button-down shirts. Jeans counted as formalwear for them (and for me too). To this day, thanks to resistance on their part and laziness on ours, we have never gotten either boy in a tie or a blazer. It's a shame, because they would look spiffy. But for this Christmas, they were attending church dressed in business casual. Despite owning five thousand hoodies, Flora put on a dress for the occasion. She's now old enough to want to look good when she's out on the town.

My extended family loaded into three separate cars and headed out for the service. Once there, we occupied a couple of pews toward the back. We did this out of habit, because getting out of a church parking lot is an unspoken but obvious pain in the ass, and also because when the kids were much smaller, we bailed early on services if they got so loud that people started to stare.

The kids weren't loud this time around. They had endured far longer stretches of uncertainty just the year before.

Colin lay down across our pew, like he was resting in the back seat during a long road trip. Rudy sat quietly and thumbed through the hymnal, looking for carols he recognized. Flora looked indifferent, mostly because we had taken her phone away. For a full hour! TALK ABOUT FUCKING TORTURE.

Same as ever, I kept a constant vigil on where we were in the program, so I knew how close we were to the end. I had appetizers I wanted to eat.

Then came the celebrant reading, bolded part mine:

> *Holy and gracious Father: In your infinite love you made us for yourself, and, when we had fallen into sin and become subject to evil and death,* **you, in your mercy, sent Jesus Christ, your only and eternal Son, to share our human nature,** *to live and die as one of us, to reconcile us to you, the God and Father of all.*

I have been unwillingly subjected to enough Scripture in my time to know the basic ins and outs of the Christian faith. Jesus died for us, God works in mysterious ways, etc. But I had never, ever thought about the idea that people were a mystery to God himself. Maybe that's not what that passage above is meant to convey, but the idea struck me all the same. I used the stubby pencil next to the collection-plate envelopes to highlight it. I had always been told God loves us, but it had never occurred to me that God found mankind all that *interesting*. But what if God, in his divine humility, doesn't see himself as superior to us but sees us as colleagues? If you're a theologian coming to assault me, please know that I'm not trying to be authoritative here. I'm barely Christian, if I'm Christian at all. It just made more sense to me that if there really was a God, he would say to himself, *What's with those people down there? What are they all about? Lemme send the boy to investigate.* What if God is *not* all-seeing and all-knowing? What if he wants to learn? And what did he find in humanity that he could not find when restricted to his own mind?

I was paying attention now. The reverend got up and delivered his sermon, in which he explained that the material and the heavenly need not be segregated from one another.

"Look around at your family, and at your friends, and at the world," he told the congregation. "It's all God. It's all holy."

I jotted down more notes in the margins of my program. Sonia caught me doing this and was baffled. *I* was baffled. I scribbled something about how epiphanies are not singular in the mind. Other thoughts mill around in there when the proverbial lightning strikes. Everything is busy in your mind. Always. Each thought lives alongside, and sometimes interacts with, many others. How it works is a mystery, but it's all valuable. It's all part of the universe and its aggregate soul. In fact, it goes beyond the universe and into planes of existence that have no physical form, if any form at all. Heaven and earth are one. Life and death are one. Everything and nothing are one. It's all one thing. It's all love, and it can never die.

Over the past year, I had gotten a crash course (pun somewhat intended) in the physiology of the brain and how it is the vital conduit to everything else that is tangible in your existence: your body, your family, your house, etc. I had not—could not, really—appreciate how lucky I was to have the brain I had. I had wasted too much time being self-conflagellatory instead. I cursed my brain for failing me that night without a warning beforehand or an explanation afterward. I shrank at the visible damage it had endured. I gnashed my teeth over its inability to bring back all of my senses unharmed.

But everyone I loved worked their asses off to save that brain. To save *me*. And they did. I was saved. Baptized in leaking spinal fluid. This was the year I discovered my life's value to others, and the realization was so immense that I felt overwhelmed by it, and I still do. I cannot fathom how so much love could exist, nor how I was lucky enough to be its recipient. It's a gorgeous, eternal mystery, and it's the mystery I'd rather spend more of my time pondering than the mystery of what exactly happened to me in that hallway.

We got home for cocktail hour. Alex wore a new fez he had bought to be extra festive. I abstained from the whiskey but not from the Cheetos. Around sevenish, we sat down in my parents' dining room. Along with the kids, I got a champagne flute filled with sparkling cranberry cider. Soda was my beer now. Mom brought out a smoked goose she had gotten from a mail-order joint in Nebraska. She carved me a slice while I guzzled cider like I was the anchor in a game of flip cup.

I took a bite. I tasted everything. I got the salt, the smoke, the fat . . . Not a single particle of flavor went undetected. This was not some miracle recovery I was staging. My time in church was not an exercise in faith healing. Something about that bird just, as a matter of good fortune, hit every taste bud that was still active on my tongue.

"Mom, I can taste this."

"Isn't it wonderful?"

"It sure as hell is."

I went back for seconds, then thirds. I regretted nothing. Geese are mean, terrible animals. They deserve to be eaten, and with great relish. I made clandestine plans to eat nothing but smoked goose from here on out. And when I was done, I laid waste to the cookie platter.

The kids put out treats and notes for Santa, laid their stockings out on the couch (my folks didn't have nails above the fireplace to hang them), and went to bed. I tucked Colin in.

"I'll see you Christmas morning!" I told him.

"No, don't say that," he insisted. "Because I wanna sleep, and if I think about Christmas I won't sleep."

"Okay."

These days, I can't wait to wake up either. I'm awfully lucky to have this brain of mine, and to use it. Some things I can never do again, true, and yet there's still so much more—by exponential orders of magnitude—that I can do that will be new!

The next morning was Christmas. A real Christmas. No hospital. No photos taped to the wall to make me feel better. No Airbnb walk-up that my family had to pretend was home. The kids tore open all their shit before I could even get a photo. Colin got a punching bag.

"Finally," he cried out, "I can hit something all I want!"

I grabbed the fancy shopping bag and handed it to Sonia. "All right," I said. "Hope this works."

She opened it and let out another spontaneous *OOOOOH*. You can tell when an *OOOOOH* is fake when you give someone a gift. This one was not.

"Oh my God, Drew, it's so nice."

"Wowie, wowie," said my mom, selling it.

"You like the snakeskin?" I asked Sonia.

"I do!"

I did a mental fistpump. Then she slung the bag over her shoulder. She hesitated for just a second. I instantly knew it was doomed.

"It's a little heavy," she said. She was more disappointed the bag wasn't quite right than I was. For my part, I knew the store had a generous return policy, as the rep had reminded me. And I knew that the love was all that mattered anyway. It's all love. It's all holy.

"That's okay," I told Sonia. All year long, I had had a nasty habit of taking gift rejections personally. Not this time. As in 2016, I was simply relieved I had been *close*. I felt no anger. No resentment. No imagined lack of respect. None of those weights. We both agreed the gift was good, regardless of whether or not Sonia actually kept it (she didn't; she returned it and bought a used designer bag that she still uses and loves). I had done my job. At long last, I had done my job. Sonia knew it. All along. She knew this would be a process. I asked her if I'd gotten any better since my accident.

"This kind of stuff takes time. I knew you were processing it and dealing with your new self. But you're the same man. You have the same heart. It could have gone so many different ways and all the wrong way, but that you are where you are now . . . It's a fricking miracle. It's a big deal. It was a tough journey and it really sucked. But we all learned things about each other. I just did the best I could. All that I could do to push on and keep the family together and get through it."

And we got through it. Together.

To celebrate, I ate half a kringle Danish on Christmas morning. To burn off that Danish, I went on a walk with Sonia, Mom, and Amanda. There are no sidewalks on my parents' street. They don't even live in a neighborhood to speak of. Their house lies along a road that connects two county highways and thus serves as an unofficial county highway itself. We walked along that thoroughfare, past a small horse stable, and then cut across the main highway to continue our stroll. To the right of the road was a great field. At the back of the field was a stone house large enough to accommodate an entire English foxhunting party. This used to be a summer estate owned by the heiress to a wealthy brass manufacturer. That heiress died and gifted the lands to the state of Connecticut, which did nothing with it. One day the house may be open for tours, but for now it remains abandoned. No one lives in it anymore, but it's still cool to look at: all finely shaped masonry, weathered stucco, ceramic chimney stacks, and slate roofs.

I grabbed an impromptu walking stick from under one of the warted trees lining the road and used it to support myself. And so I could feel like a wizard. The walk was getting longer than any of us had expected, but I didn't want to stop. I couldn't. I wanted to keep putting one foot in front of the other.

We had to navigate a steep slope to get a better view of the house. I took Mom's hand and we ducked under an aged wooden gate and hiked up toward the field, supporting each other to keep ourselves upright. We got closer to the mansion, walking along a path cut through stalks of wild wheat. The mansion was grand from a distance but frayed and cramped up close. Needed a little bit of love. Maybe a few ceiling fans. And an infinity pool. But with a little extra care, it would make a fine home.

We went back to my parents' house and Dad made a fire. My folks' fireplace has a hearth that sits at waist level, so you can see the flames from every vantage point in the room. I got close to the fire, as was customary for me. I grabbed the andirons and shuffled the logs around so that the charred parts faced away from the stack and the virgin parts of the wood could catch flame. I heard the flames chugging oxygen as they stretched up toward the flue. I leaned in and gave the fire a sniff. I could smell the smoke, just as I had been able to taste it the night before. Once again, the world had found a sweet spot inside my brain at the most romantic possible moment. I looked down at the embers and their deep heat, glowing with such heft that they beckoned you closer to watch them burn. Long after the flames died down, those embers would remain glowing and alive.

I'm a little different now. I get tired easily. My battery drains faster. Alarm clocks are still a 50/50 proposition for me. I've lost some things. But you cannot lose what has already been. I wasn't "better," but in other ways, perhaps I was. For so long, I believed that nothing good could ever have come from this. But that isn't how things work. To live on, you have to *make* the good happen. A different life need not be a worse one. You have to decide if you're the lucky one or not. Why live on otherwise?

I was the lucky one. I was the last to understand it. Little Colin, who nearly died at nine days old, still didn't grasp how lucky *he* had been to survive. Carter, resting lazily back at my in-laws' house in Maryland . . . he didn't know how lucky *he* had been to be pulled out of a shelter three years prior. I will never know what Carter's early life was like. I don't even know his real age. I can only speculate on the potential traumas he may have endured as a stray dog or as an unwanted pet. But I don't regret saving him. Ever. And I'll always love him, even though there are things about him I can never, ever know. Love means accepting each other's mysteries.

It's those inexplicable facets of love that give it an eternal sheen. The people who saved me? They had always been saving me, and they're still saving me to this day. I'm still processing this—in ways both conscious and unconscious—and I suppose I always will. But that processing is more of a gift than a burden. It's a reminder of what I have, and a reminder to preserve my family's memory of me as my own. We are each other's memories. We are each other's brains. We are, forever, rewiring one another.

I kept staring at the fire. Hearing it. Smelling it. I'm not the man I was, but I'm still in there. Still burning bright.

EPILOGUE

Defector Media officially launched on September 12, 2020. Staffers included me, **Barry Petchesky, Samer Kalaf, Lauren Theisen, Kelsey McKinney, Chris Thompson, Diana Moskovitz, Albert Burneko, Patrick Redford, David Roth,** and nine other former Deadspin writers and editors. We were starting a new, self-owned media company, in the middle of a pandemic, without any of the original seed money. We weren't gonna be able to pay ourselves any money at first. If Defector failed, we wouldn't be able to pay ourselves at all.

But Defector didn't fail.

Jorge Corona and **Kiran Chitanvis** left G/O Media shortly after the entire Deadspin staff did. They both now work as independent filmmakers. **Victor Jeffreys,** who was unceremoniously fired by G/O Media on New Year's Eve of 2019 after enduring harassment from upper management, is now an all-purpose fixer for the world at large instead of merely for one company. **Bobby Silverman,** the man whose need for cigarettes indirectly saved my brain, is currently a freelance journalist. **Gabe Fernandez** currently writes for CBS Sports. **Matt Ufford** is now a director at ESPN. **Byrd Leavell** is still my agent. **Will Leitch** is now a columnist for Major League Baseball and a contributing editor to *New York* magazine.

After getting laid off by G/O Media, **Susie Banikarim** joined Vice News as their executive vice president. She still lives in New York, as do **Megan Greenwell** and her husband, **Dr. David Heller.** Megan, godmother to Defector, served as the editor of Wired.com before resigning in April 2021, citing burnout. David remains an internist at Mount Sinai and was one of the many doctors and staffers enlisted into extended duty when COVID-19 overran that hospital, New York City, and the United States as a whole. Mine is far from the only life he's saved.

In late 2020, I got a form letter from **Dr. John Caridi**, announcing that he was leaving his post at Mt. Sinai. Dr. Caridi now works as chief of the neurosurgical spine division at the UTHealth Neurosciences Spine Center in Houston, TX. If *you* ever pull a Humpty Dumpty on a bar floor, and you live in Texas, I cannot recommend seeing Dr. Caridi strongly enough.

Dr. Michael Morikawa remains a clinical audiologist at Georgetown Hospital. I still go to him for regular Rondo tune-ups. I also still go to **Dr. Kent** regularly as well and would happily recommend him to anyone, deaf or otherwise.

Howard got married in Mexico City in October 2020 and lives with his wife on the Upper West Side of Manhattan. His sister, **Erica,** lives with her husband and two children in suburban Connecticut. **Jesse** and his family, also living in NYC, got a new dog named Archie for Christmas 2020. If Archie is anything like our Christmas gift dog, Jesse is in for happy times.

My sister, **Amanda,** is director of counseling at a prep school and lives with her husband and three kids in a house roughly 45 minutes away from **Mom** and **Dad.** Mom is still her glamorous self. Dad quit drinking shortly after Mom did, and has since taken up eating ice cream in admirable quantities. My brother, **Alex,** lives in

New Hampshire with his two children and still works as in-house counsel to a health technology company. I believe he still owns the Christmas fez.

Flora, Rudy, and **Colin** all attended virtual school throughout the entirety of the 2020–2021 year. Flora has already told us that when the pandemic is over, she's blowing this joint and never coming back. I can't blame her.

Sonia's preschool temporarily closed during the pandemic, but my wife isn't the type to let a global death plague stand in the way of being productive. She now does paintings on commission and plans to return to teaching in the fall of 2021.

Carter is still a very good dog. He's so mellowed out these days, he barely gets off the couch. It's like a second husband lives here.

In the middle of quarantine, while I was bored to death, I got heavy into the idea of buying a karaoke machine. I hadn't done any karaoke since my accident, and I wanted to make up for lost tunes. I figured I could keep the machine in the basement, where more perceptive ears wouldn't be able to hear me rocking out to Oasis. I told Sonia about my idea. This was her response:

"If you buy a karaoke machine, I really may have to divorce you."

I never bought it.

ACKNOWLEDGMENTS

Matthew Benjamin was the editor in charge of this book. He's the best book editor I've ever had, and by a substantial margin. The copy editor was Hilary Roberts and the production editor was Abby Oladipo. Both these women had to deal with my all-caps fetish and did so with ÉLAN. Megan Greenwell, David Heller, Kelsey McKinney, and my wife also contributed vital edits. Matthew Martin handled the legal review. Jen Valero designed the interior layout of the book and made the copy fly. Pete Garceau designed the cover. It's a great fucking cover. Nothing more fun than writing a book and then being handed this kind of cover. It's like getting an award.

I remain indebted to everyone in this book not merely because they saved my life, but because they were also willing to be interviewed at length by me—during a pandemic, no less—so that I could write it. If they ever find themselves in similarly dire straits, I hope that I'll be as dutiful and as generous as they were when *I* was in deep shit. I owe all of them that, and more. But of course, I pray that none of my friends and loved ones ever experience such travails to begin with. To this day, I still feel bad they had to endure all of that. So to them, I just wanna say: Thank you. And sorry about the whole hemorrhage thing. I won't do it again.